Eating Disorders

Editor: Tracy Biram

Volume 390

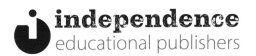
independence
educational publishers

First published by Independence Educational Publishers

The Studio, High Green

Great Shelford

Cambridge CB22 5EG

England

© Independence 2021

Copyright

Photocopy licence

ISBN-13: 978 1 86168 848 4

Printed in Great Britain

Zenith Print Group

Contents

Introduction

Eating Disorders is Volume 390 in the **issues** series. The aim of the series is to offer current, diverse information about important issues in our world, from a UK perspective.

ABOUT EATING DISORDERS

Approximately 1.25 million people in the UK have an eating disorder. Problems with eating can start at any age, but mostly start in the teenage years. This book explores why eating disorders may develop, the different types of eating problems and disorders, and what can be done to tackle disordered eating.

OUR SOURCES

Titles in the **issues** series are designed to function as educational resource books, providing a balanced overview of a specific subject.

The information in our books is comprised of facts, articles and opinions from many different sources, including:

♦ Newspaper reports and opinion pieces

♦ Website factsheets

♦ Magazine and journal articles

♦ Statistics and surveys

♦ Government reports

♦ Literature from special interest groups.

A NOTE ON CRITICAL EVALUATION

Because the information reprinted here is from a number of different sources, readers should bear in mind the origin of the text and whether the source is likely to have a particular bias when presenting information (or when conducting their research). It is hoped that, as you read about the many aspects of the issues explored in this book, you will critically evaluate the information presented.

It is important that you decide whether you are being presented with facts or opinions. Does the writer give a biased or unbiased report? If an opinion is being expressed, do you agree with the writer? Is there potential bias to the 'facts' or statistics behind an article?

ASSIGNMENTS

In the back of this book, you will find a selection of assignments designed to help you engage with the articles you have been reading and to explore your own opinions. Some tasks will take longer than others and there is a mixture of design, writing and research-based activities that you can complete alone or in a group.

FURTHER RESEARCH

At the end of each article we have listed its source and a website that you can visit if you would like to conduct your own research. Please remember to critically evaluate any sources that you consult and consider whether the information you are viewing is accurate and unbiased.

Useful Websites

www.bjfm.co.uk

www.creativeyouthnetwork.org.uk

www.digital.nhs.uk

www.FLEXEBEE.co.uk

www.independent.co.uk

www.inews.co.uk

www.joe.co.uk

www.liverpoolecho.co.uk

wtww.mind.org.uk

www.newbridge-health.org.uk

www.northernhealthcare.org.uk

www.oxfordhealth.nhs.uk

www.rhitririon.com

www.taliacecchele.com

www.telegraph.co.uk

www.theguardian.com

www.thelondoncentre.co.uk

www.themix.org.uk

www.wearencs.com

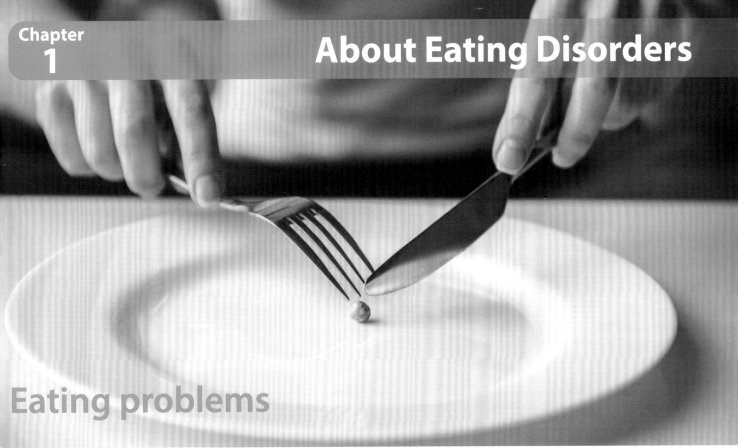

Eating problems

What is an eating problem?

An eating problem is any relationship with food that you find difficult.

Many people think that someone with an eating problem will be over or underweight. People might also think that certain weights are linked to certain eating problems. Neither of these points are true.

Anyone can experience eating problems. This is regardless of age, gender, weight or background.

Food plays a significant part in our lives. Most of us will spend time thinking about what we eat. Sometimes you might:

♦ have cravings

♦ eat more than usual

♦ lose your appetite

♦ try to eat healthier.

Changing your eating habits like this every now and again is normal.

But if you feel like food and eating is taking over your life, it may become a problem.

What's the difference between an eating problem and an eating disorder?

♦ **An eating disorder is a medical diagnosis.** This diagnosis is based on your eating patterns and includes medical tests on your weight, blood and body mass index (BMI). See our page on diagnosed eating disorders for more information.

♦ **An eating problem is any relationship with food that you find difficult.** This can be just as hard to live with as a diagnosed eating disorder.

What's it like to have an eating problem?

If you have an eating problem, there are many ways that it can affect how you feel or behave. The way you eat, and how you think about food, may be one of the most noticeable effects.

How might I behave if I have an eating problem?

If you have an eating problem, you might be familiar with some of the following behaviours.

You might:

♦ restrict the amount of food you eat

♦ eat more than you need, or feel out of control when you eat

♦ eat regularly in secret or have a fear of eating in public

♦ feel very anxious about eating or digesting food

♦ eat in response to difficult emotions without feeling physically hungry

♦ stick to a rigid set of diet rules or certain foods

♦ feel anxious and upset if you have to eat something else

♦ do things to get rid of what you eat, sometimes known as purging

♦ feel disgusted at the idea of eating certain foods

♦ eat things that aren't really food, such as dirt, soap or paint

♦ feel scared of certain types of food

♦ think about food and eating a lot, even all the time

♦ compare your body to other people's and think a lot about its shape or size

- check, test and weigh your body very often
- base your self-worth on your weight, or whether you pass your checks and tests.

'Food was like poison to me. It resembled all the negativity in my life. It made me feel weighed down by impurity, dirtiness, ugliness and selfishness. My body shape made me miserable and I spent all day everyday thinking about how great life would be if I was skinny.'

How might eating problems affect my life?

Eating problems are not just about food. They can be about difficult things and painful feelings. You may be finding these hard to express, face or resolve.

Focusing on food can be a way of hiding these feelings and problems, even from yourself. Eating problems can affect you in lots of ways.

You might feel:

- depressed and anxious
- tired a lot of the time
- ashamed or guilty
- scared of other people finding out.

You might find that:

- it's hard to concentrate on your work, studies or hobbies
- controlling food or eating has become the most important thing in your life
- it's hard to be spontaneous, to travel or to go anywhere new
- your appearance is changing or has changed
- you are bullied or teased about food and eating
- you develop short- or long-term physical health problems
- you want to avoid socialising, dates and restaurants or eating in public
- you have to drop out of school or college, leave work or stop doing things you enjoy.

With friends, family or other people, you might feel that:

- you're distant from those who don't know how you feel, or who are upset they can't do more to help
- they focus a lot on the effect eating problems can have on your body
- they only think you have a problem if your body looks different to how they think it should be
- they sometimes comment on your appearance in ways you find difficult
- they don't really understand how complicated things are for you.

'I wish people would move away from stereotypes and understand that eating disorders are not only to do with weight, but thoughts, feelings and behaviours – regardless of the number a scale shows, and regardless of physical appearance.'

How do I know if it's a problem?

As it may feel like part of your everyday life, you might be unsure if your issue with food and eating is a problem. But if your relationship with food and eating is affecting your life, you can seek help. It doesn't matter how much you weigh or what your body looks like.

Some people don't seek help because they think their problem is not serious enough. Sometimes they do not feel 'ill enough' to have an eating problem.

It's also possible to have problems with eating and keep them hidden. Sometimes this can be for very long time.

'I never looked "ill". When I read about eating disorders it was always girls with acute anorexia. Because that wasn't me, I felt like my behaviour was just a bizarre quirk I'd made up.'

Eating problems and other mental health problems

Many people with eating problems also have other mental health problems. Some common experiences include:

- depression
- anxiety
- obsessive-compulsive disorders
- phobias of certain foods
- issues with self-esteem and body image
- forms of self-harm – you may see your eating problem as a form of self-harm, or may hurt yourself in other ways too
- body dysmorphic disorder, which is an anxiety disorder linked to body image.

Food is one of many mediums through which anxiety, depression or obsessive-compulsive behaviours can be expressed.

'My eating disorder has always gone hand in hand with depression and anxiety in such a way that they haven't felt like distinct, discrete illnesses but like one issue.'

Eating disorders

The subtle signs and symptoms.

By Rebecca Hallworth

When we think of the term 'eating disorder' we often associate it with an individual who starves themselves, but it has many applications. An eating disorder is an unhealthy attitude towards food. It can involve eating too much, or eating too little, or becoming obsessed with your weight and body. Some eating disorders may be easier to see than others, some you might not be able to spot at all from simply looking at an individual. In this blog, we explore the types of eating disorders and how you may be able to identify and help someone who is struggling with their eating:

Types of eating disorders

Approximately 1.25 million people in the UK have an eating disorder. Eating disorders are a collection of conditions which include anorexia, bulimia, binge eating and OSFED. It may be surprising to hear that OSFED (other specified feeding or eating disorder) is the most common, followed by binge eating disorder and then bulimia. Anorexia is the least common. Here are some of the common eating disorders defined:

Anorexia Nervosa – keeping your body weight as low as you can by not eating, exercising too much, or a combination of the two.

Bulimia – People with bulimia will eat a lot of food in a very short amount of time (binging) and are then deliberately sick or they may overuse laxatives. They may also restrict what they eat or do too much exercise to prevent gaining weight.

Binge Eating Disorder (BED) – when you regularly lose control of your eating, eat large portions of food all at once until you feel uncomfortably full, and then feel upset or guilty.

Other Specified Feeding or Eating Disorder (OSFED) – Similarly to the conditions listed above OSFED is a mental illness that is not only about the way in which someone consumes food, but also their thoughts and feelings towards food and their self-image. A person with OSFED may not exactly exhibit all the behaviours associated with anorexia, bulimia or binge eating disorder, but it does not mean it is a less serious illness.

What are the signs of an eating disorder?

It can be very difficult to recognise whether you or someone you know has developed an eating disorder. Not all symptoms exactly match those for anorexia, bulimia or binge eating disorder and many people may be suffering with an eating disorder but still maintaining a consistent weight.

Dramatic weight loss or gain, are signs of eating disorders, but other symptoms include worrying about weight and body shape – talking about it excessively, eating very little food or too much food, avoiding eating with others, making yourself sick, lying about what you have eaten or your weight, taking laxatives after you eat and dramatic weight loss.

But what about the signs we miss?

Extreme exercising: It is hard to tell whether someone is excessively exercising. If exercise takes over someone's life and they panic or become distressed if they miss a workout, this could be a sign.

Fear of eating in public: Feeling shy when eating in public is common, but it can also be an indicator of an eating disorder. Individuals can develop a high level of anxiety associated with eating. Sometimes people believe that others are watching and judging them.

Eating rituals: Cutting food up into small pieces and arranging food in a particular way is a method used to disguise how little someone has eaten.

Dental issues and dry skin: People with bulimia often purge and some take laxatives. This causes severe dehydration. Purging also causes dental problems due to stomach acid. Anorexia also causes tooth loss due to lack of nutrients causing the bones to become weak.

Wearing baggy clothes: Baggy clothes are often used to hide weight loss amongst people suffering with anorexia.

Excessive interest in what other people eat: Asking people what they ate/eat or asking them to describe what their meal tastes like in detail are both signs of an eating disorder.

Food habits: Using large quantities of seasoning on food and mixing uncommon combinations of sweet with savoury, drinking excessive amounts of tea and coffee, continuously chewing gum, hoarding food and hiding food wrappers can all be signs of an eating disorder.

Food obsession: It is common for people with an eating disorder to have an intense interest in food. This can result in a collection of recipes, cookbooks, menus and kitchen utensils or even watching programmes about food and looking at pictures of food. Claiming to follow a vegan, gluten-free or a low-calorie diet can also be a cover for an eating disorder.

Getting help

Recovery from an eating disorder is different for everyone. Treatment depends on the type of eating disorder you have. The first step is to speak to someone and let your GP know. Your GP can refer you to a specialist who will be responsible for your care.

If you are worried about someone else, then you should approach the conversation with them sensitively. People with an eating disorder are often secretive and defensive. Let them know that you are there for them and encourage them to seek support from their GP.

www.northernhealthcare.org.uk

Eating disorders - what types of eating disorders exist ?

Eating disorders can be emotionally and physically depleting conditions. According to eating disorder charity Beat, at least 1.25 million people in the UK suffer from these, with up to 6.4% of the population showing signs of developing the conditions.

Much more attention is given to eating disorders than has historically been the case, meaning more work is being done to help cure those who suffer from the problems.

However, there are a variety of different eating disorders, and each affects its victims differently. This article takes a brief look at the symptoms of some of the most common eating disorders.

Before going further, it is worth mentioning some of the avenues of support available if you (or someone you know) wishes to get help with an eating disorder. It is recommended that you speak with a GP about the problem so that you can be referred to the appropriate specialists.

Different eating disorders

The four most common eating disorders in the UK, in descending order, are:

- Other Specified Feeding or Eating Disorder (OSFED)
- Binge Eating Disorder (BED)
- Bulimia
- Anorexia Nervosa

While these are the most common types of eating disorders, various other types do exist. For example, pica is an eating disorder characterised by consumption of non-nutritious matter such as ice or hair, and diabulimia is an eating disorder that can only affect people with Type 1 diabetes.

Anorexia Nervosa

Anorexia nervosa is an eating disorder where people try and keep their weight as low as possible. This is normally achieved by not eating enough food or exercising far too much.

Many victims of anorexia tend to think they are overweight or even obese despite being hugely underweight. It is most common in younger women, normally onsetting during the mid-teens.

Symptoms of anorexia nervosa can include an unusually low BMI in adults, lower than expected weight and height in under-18s, and frequent use of appetite suppressants. Missing meals, describing yourself as overweight when you objectively aren't, and physical problems (normally hair loss, dry skin, or light-headedness) are also associated symptoms.

Very frequently, victims of anorexia will induce vomiting in an attempt to reduce their weight. This can lead to a serious worsening of side effects, exacerbating conditions like malnutrition and dehydration.

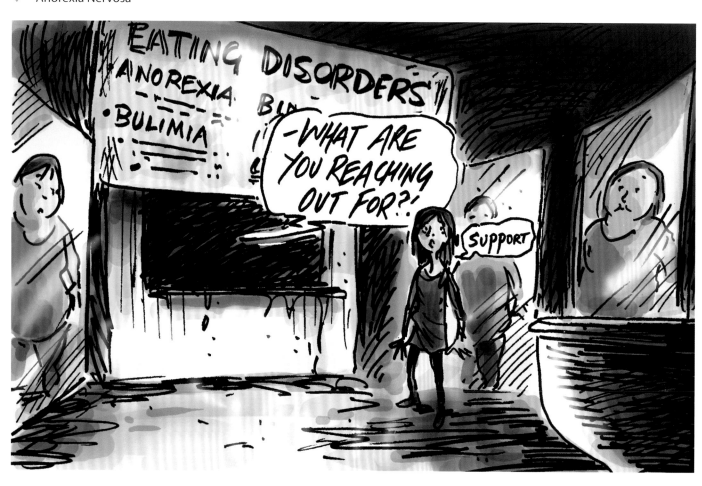

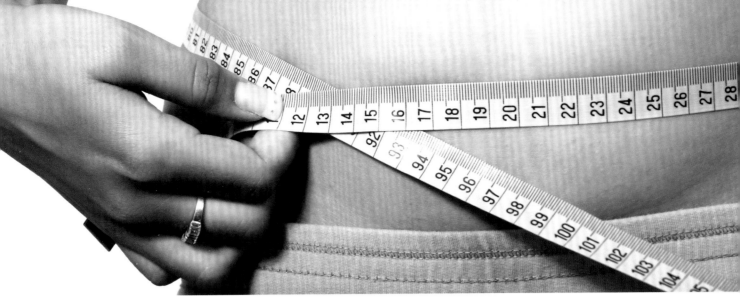

Bulimia

Bulimia and anorexia often get conflated or confused with one another, because both involve a fear of gaining weight and deliberate inducing of vomit.

However, the two are different disorders entirely. Bulimia is characterised as a disorder where people go through periods of out of control binge-eating, followed by periods of intense fear over the thought of gaining weight, ending with attempts to try and lose weight through methods such as vomiting or excessive exercise.

These three things are the main symptoms, but people with bulimia often also have mood changes. The fear that bulimic people experience over the thought of being overweight is an important difference between bulimia and anorexia, since fixing a fear is a much different process to correcting misconceptions someone has with the way they perceive themselves in the world.

Binge eating disorder

Binge eating is a symptom of bulimia, but binge eating disorder is a category of its own. BED, as it is also known, doesn't involve fear of being overweight, misperceptions about one's actual weight, or any extreme attempts to fix the problem such as excessive exercise.

Rather, people with BED eat large portions of food at one time regularly until they are uncomfortably full or feel ill. This often results in feelings of intense guilt or upset. Binges are typically planned, food stockpiled for them, and are often done very quickly in secret, when someone isn't physically hungry.

It is particularly prevalent in the late teens and early twenties.

Other specified feeding or eating disorders

The largest individual category of eating disorders are other specified feeding or eating disorders (OSFED). These are also serious eating disorders, but present in different ways to standard disorders like anorexia nervosa. Some of the most common OSFED diagnoses are:

- ◆ **Atypical Anorexia:** a condition the same as anorexia nervosa, but the victim's weight stays within a normal range
- ◆ **Purging Disorder:** a disorder comprised entirely of the use of laxatives or emetics to alter weight, yet isn't part of the binging/purging cycle in conditions such as bulimia

- ◆ **Low Frequency / Limited Duration Bulimia Nervosa:** a type of bulimia wherein all the standard symptoms are present, but the cycles of over-eating and purging are of a shorter duration than would be expected
- ◆ **Low Frequency / Limited Duration Binge Eating Disorder:** like above, all the symptoms of binge eating disorder are present, but periods of binge eating do not take place over the same duration as would normally be expected
- ◆ **Night Eating Syndrome:** a disorder that sees the person suffering from it repeatedly eating at night – normally after waking up during the night or binge eating a lot of food after the evening meal

It is sometimes more difficult to assess if someone is suffering from an OSFED. While something like purging disorder can clearly be identified as a problem, things such as night eating syndrome can sometimes be written off as quirky behaviours.

If episodes of bulimia are short, they could be viewed as 'phases' that someone will grow out of, or someone with concerns about being anorexic might be written off as attention-seeking because they are in a normal weight range.

This is why it is important to seek medical advice as soon as possible if you think you might be suffering from an eating disorder.

Further reading:

The NHS website has information about many types of eating disorders, including the treatments that are available and causes of them: www.nhs.uk

The charity Beat, as well as providing confidential advice hotlines, has a lot of information on their website about eating disorders and their symptoms: www.beateatingdisorders.org.uk

17 June 2020

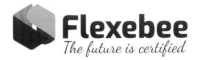

www.FLEXEBEE.co.uk

Disordered eating and how to break the cycle

By Talia Cecchele, Registered Dietitian

Unlike eating disorders which are classified using *The Diagnostic and Statistical Manual of Mental Disorders* (DSM-5), disordered eating has no official definition. Generally, it refers to disturbed and abnormal eating behaviours which might include skipping meals, restrictive dieting or rigid rules around eating e.g. removing a major food group from the diet.

The eating disorders charity Beat estimates that approximately 1.25 million people in the UK have a diagnosed eating disorder falling under four categories: anorexia nervosa (AN), bulimia nervosa (BN), binge eating disorder (BED) and Other Specified Feeding or Eating Disorder (OSFED). It is thought that in reality it could be double that amount as many people do not seek help or have access to it so are not captured in the figures. We could speculate that a large majority of people in the UK are engaging in disordered eating behaviour but it is unclear in the research and difficult to estimate due to the lack of an official definition and criteria.

Eating disorders are complex and there is no one single reason why someone might develop an eating disorder. Environment and social factors are just some of the reasons that can combine to influence someone's chance. With the rise in diet culture, social media and increased food availability (and therefore dietary choice) I believe our modern society can increase a person's risk.

It is hard to believe that anyone has a normal relationship with food when dieting and engaging in disordered eating is the new normal, but many of us definitely do. Having a normal relationship with food includes four key components to eating: regular eating, diet variety (not cutting out food groups or particular foods unnecessarily), being flexible with food choices and eating with enjoyment.

While it is most common among young women, disordered eating can affect anyone of any age, gender or race. You are more likely to be affected if there is a family history of eating disorders or mental health illness, you have been criticised for your eating or the way you look, there is a pressure to look thin (for example models, athletes or ballet dancers), you have anxiety or low self esteem or have experienced trauma. We also know that there is a link between social media use and greater body image concerns and disordered eating (Holland & Tiggemann, 2016).

How do you know if disordered eating is becoming a bigger problem?

Many people with disordered eating will meet criteria for a clinically diagnosed eating disorder, but having unhealthy eating behaviours doesn't necessarily mean that this will morph into an eating disorder. Some of the warning signs include:

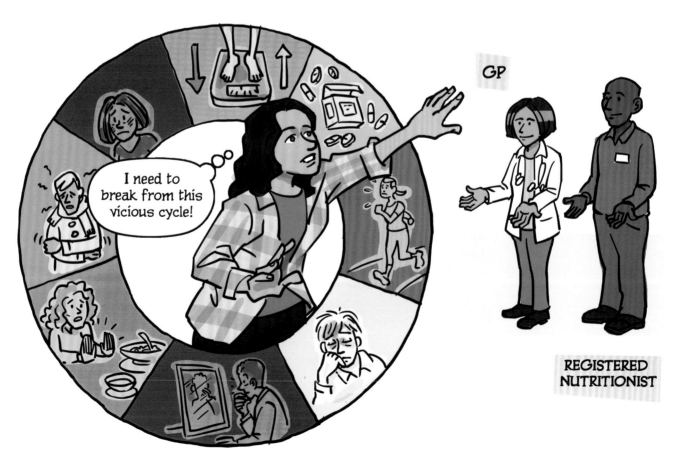

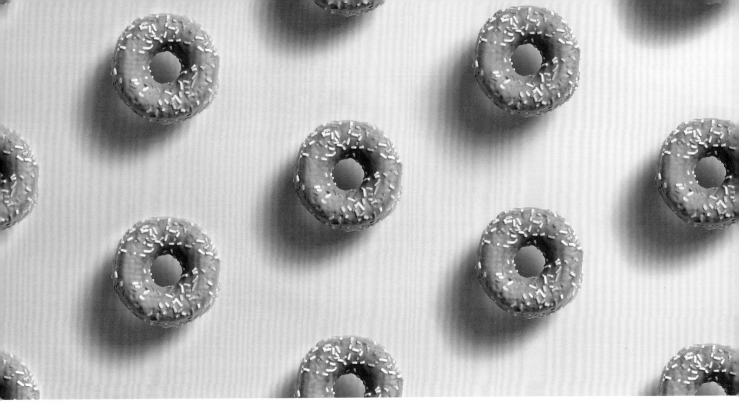

- Spending a lot of time worrying about how you look and what you eat
- Avoiding social events with food
- Eating very little food
- Counting calories or measuring food obsessively
- Very strict dietary rules
- Deliberately engaging in behaviours that alter your weight and digestion including vomiting, laxative use, taking diet pills or excessive exercise
- Feeling cold, dizzy and tired all the time
- Digestive issues including IBS type symptoms
- Losing weight or gaining weight quickly
- Losing your period or irregular periods

How does this affect your health?

Many people who engage in disordered eating either minimise these behaviours or do not realise the effect it could have on their physical and mental health. It is terrifying to see serious side effects often glorified by weight loss companies. Disordered eating can pose serious health concerns including risk of obesity, underweight or eating disorders, long-term gastrointestinal issues, osteoporosis, fertility issues, low heart rate and blood pressure and impact on mental health including anxiety and depression.

What can you do break the cycle of disordered eating

I recommend making an appointment with your GP to check your physical health before making any significant changes to your eating and lifestyle. I would advise anyone who has severely restricted their diet or engaged in extreme compensatory behaviours (vomiting, laxative use or excessive exercise) to consult a Registered Dietitian or Registered Nutritionist for advice such as, us here at the Rhitrition Clinic where we have a team of professionals to help. The first steps towards dietary changes would be to eat regular meals and snacks and adding a variety of foods back into your diet. It can be helpful to take a break off social media or to unfollow unhelpful accounts, and reach out for help from friends and family as challenging disordered eating can be harder that we think so the more support the better.

What to do if disordered eating worsens

The first port of call is to speak to your GP to see what services are available locally or to get a referral to a practitioner who specialises in eating disorders. At the Rhitrition Clinic in London, we have a team of Registered Dietitians and Nutritionists that are trained to help people suffering from eating disorders and disordered eating. You can also call the Beat helpline on 0808 801 0677 or head to their website for helpful resources for both people suffering from disordered eating and their family/carers.

What support can you give to those you are worried about?

It can be difficult to know what to do and what to say if you are concerned about a friend. Let them know that you are worried, ask how they are feeling and how you can help. I would advise anyone to encourage their friend or family member to seek help and make an appointment with their GP or call the Beat helpline. It is important to avoid talking about weight, shape, food or diets in front of them and to be a role model when it comes to meal times. It is also important to remember not to blame or accuse someone of their eating behaviours - no one chooses to have an eating disorder. For more information about how to help, head to the Beat website.

More than quarter of young women have possible eating disorder, major study finds

'Shocking' findings suggest eating disorders 'may be an even bigger issue than previously thought,' says charity.

By Maya Oppenheim, Women's Correspondent

More than one in four young women have a potential eating disorder as experts warn the 'shocking' new figures demonstrate specialist health services need to be substantially expanded.

The Health Survey for England, which polled 8,205 adults in 2019, discovered one in six adults in England has a possible eating disorder.

While four per cent said anxieties about food impinged their ability to work, carry out personal responsibilities or have a social life.

Some 28 per cent of women who were aged between 16 and 24 and 27 per cent of women from 25 to 34 had a potential eating disorder. Researchers found around one in eight male adults have a possible eating disorder.

Andrew Radford, chief executive of Beat, the leading eating disorder charity in the UK, told *The Independent* the new figures show 'stronger action' is required to make sure everyone who is suffering from an eating disorder or is at risk of doing so receives support and treatment.

He added: 'These figures are shocking and highlight that eating disorders may be an even bigger issue than previously thought.

'The additional government funding being provided for eating disorder services, is very welcome news, but in children's services it appears to be too often diverted elsewhere, while for adults the amount simply needs to be increased and released more quickly.

'The finding that people living with obesity are more likely to be affected by an eating disorder raises two important points. Firstly, the government must change tack to ensure its anti-obesity campaigns do not increase the risk to people with eating disorders.'

Mr Radford also called for urgent measures to be taken to reverse the 'chronic underfunding' and dearth of binge eating disorder services.

He added: 'It is essential that services are significantly expanded so that anyone affected, from any diagnosis, can get the help they need at the very earliest opportunity.'

It is estimated that 1.25 million people in the UK have an eating disorder — such as bulimia and anorexia nervosa — with the majority of those being female.

The figure also includes those who binge eat, which can lead to being overweight.

The research found 27 per cent of men and 29 per cent of women were obese in 2019 — far higher than the 14 per cent of men and 17 per cent of women in 1994.

The research found the amount of adults with diabetes has trebled in the last 25 years - rising from three per cent of men and two per cent of women in 1994 to nine per cent and six per cent respectively in 2019.

Researchers discovered 68 per cent of men and 60 per cent of women were overweight or obese in 2019, which is a sharp surge from the 58 per cent of men and 49 per cent of women in 1994.

A report recently shared exclusively with *The Independent* found eight in 10 women suffering from eating disorders are fearful for their own safety during the second national lockdown which took place in November.

Altum Health, a London-based practice of psychologists, said there had been a surge in people with eating disorders ringing for support after the UK's coronavirus lockdown. It called for urgent support for those suffering from such disorders in the wake of current nationwide measures to contain coronavirus.

15 December 2020

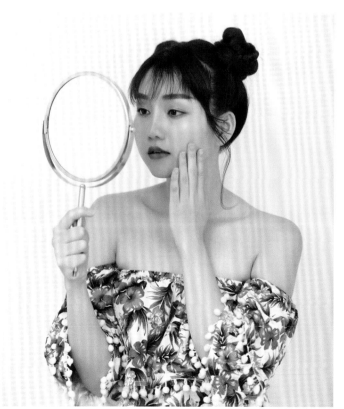

Health Survey for England 2019: Eating disorders

An extract.

An eating disorder is related to having an unhealthy attitude towards food. This can involve eating too much or too little, being obsessed with weight or body shape, changes in mood, excessive exercise, having strict habits or routines around food or purging after eating. People with eating disorders often experience psychological distress as well as physical complications, such as feeling tired or dizzy, problems with digestion or an absence of menstruation in women and girls. The most common types of eating disorders are anorexia nervosa, bulimia nervosa, binge eating disorder and other specified food or eating disorder.

Anorexia nervosa is characterised by a significantly low body weight. This is accompanied by a persistent pattern of behaviours to prevent restoration of normal weight; for example, by reducing calorie intake, purging, and excessive exercise. Having a low body weight is central to self-evaluation and can be inaccurately perceived to be a normal or excessive weight.

Bulimia nervosa is characterised by frequent, recurrent episodes of binge eating. This is accompanied by repeated compensatory behaviours at preventing weight gain, such as self-induced vomiting, misuse of laxatives, excessive exercise. The individual is preoccupied with body shape or weight. People with bulimia nervosa may maintain a more normal body weight, but can also have severe physical complications.

Why are eating disorders important?

Approximately 1.25 million people in the UK have an eating disorder. It is estimated that between 10% and 25% of those with an eating disorder are men. Most eating disorders develop during the late teens to the mid-twenties. However, it is not uncommon for eating disorders to affect people of all ages.

The SCOFF screening test

During the last year...

... have you lost more than one stone in a 3 month period?

... have you made yourself be sick because you felt uncomfortably full?

... did you worry you had lost control over how much you eat?

... did you believe yourself to be fat when others said you were too thin?

...would you say food dominated your life?

Yes/No

In this report, a positive screening for a possible eating disorder is a SCOFF score of two or more. Using the SCOFF screening tool does not allow for different types of eating disorders to be specifically identified

Having an eating disorder is linked to long term health implications including obesity, poor functioning of the body, infertility, stunted growth, brittle bones, damage to internal organs and low levels of essential vitamins. Having an eating disorder can also manifest psychologically including sleep problems, difficulty concentrating, feeling down, loss of interest in others and obsessive behaviours. It is common that eating disorders can occur alongside mental health conditions such as depression, personality disorders and substance abuse. Often an eating disorder is one of several conditions that is having a significant impact upon individuals and their quality of life.

The charity Beat Eating Disorders estimated the costs of eating disorders in 2015 based on a prevalence at the time of 600,000 to 725,000. They reported 'an annual direct financial burden of between £2.6 billion and £3.1 billion on sufferers and carers, total treatment costs to the NHS of between £3.9 billion and £4.6 billion (and, potentially, a further £0.9 billion to £1.1 billion of private treatment costs) and lost income to the economy of between £6.8 billion and £8 billion'.

The number of hospital admissions for individuals who had an eating disorder was 4,849 in 2007/08 (admissions of 4,440 women and 409 men). In 2018/19, this had increased to 17,396 admissions of women (7,554 related to anorexia, 3,831 bulimia nervosa, 6,011 another eating disorder) and 1,709 admissions of men (450 related to anorexia, 402 bulimia, 857 other eating disorder). These are not equivalent to the number of patients with an eating disorder in England as people can have more than one hospital admission.

Prevalence of screening positive for a possible eating disorder

Positive screening for possible eating disorder, by age and sex

In 2019, 16% of adults aged 16 and over had a score of 2 or more on the SCOFF scale, so screened positive for a possible eating disorder. This included 4% of adults who reported that their feelings about food had a significant negative impact on their lives.

As explained in the Introduction to this report, survey estimates are subject to a margin of error. It is likely that the proportion of adults in the population who screened positive for a possible eating disorder is between 15% and 17%, and the proportion of adults in the population who reported that their feelings about food had a significant negative impact on their life is between 4% and 5%.

Women were more likely than men to screen positive for a possible eating disorder (19% and 13%, respectively). The proportion who reported a possible eating disorder varied between age groups, following a slightly different pattern among men and women, although higher among women for all age groups under 65. Among women, prevalence was highest in those aged under 35 (28% of those aged 16 to 24, 27% aged 25 to 34). Prevalence thereafter declined broadly

Figure 1: Screened positive for possible eating disorder in past year, by age and sex

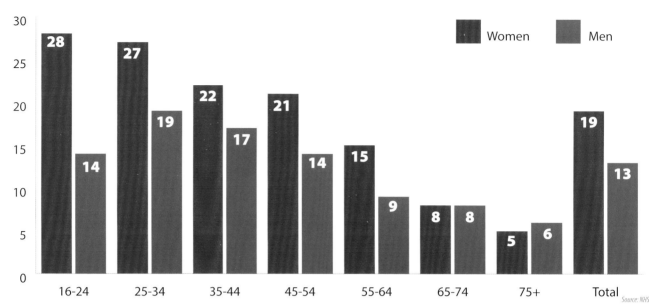

Women ■ Men

Age group	Women	Men
16-24	28	14
25-34	27	19
35-44	22	17
45-54	21	14
55-64	15	9
65-74	8	8
75+	5	6
Total	19	13

Source: NHS Digital

in line with age and was lowest among those aged 75 and over (5%). Among men, prevalence was highest among those aged 25 to 34 (19%), and then also declined with age to 6% of those aged 75 and over.

Women were more likely than men to report that their feelings about food had a significant negative impact on their lives (5% and 3%, respectively). The proportion of adults who reported such an impact on their lives differed between age groups. It was highest in those aged 35 to 44 years (7%) and lowest in those aged 75 and over (1%).

Health service use and possible eating disorder

GP visits in last year, by whether screened positive for a possible eating disorder

Adults who screened positive for a possible eating disorder were more likely to have seen a GP in the last 12 months than adults who did not screen positive (82% and 74% respectively). Among those who screened positive for a possible eating disorder, 87% of women had seen a GP

compared to 76% of men. These patterns were also seen among those who reported that their feelings about food had a significant negative impact on their lives: 87% of these adults had seen a GP in the last 12 months, including 83% of men and 90% of women.

Adults with a possible eating disorder were also likely to have visited their GP more often than other adults. 39% of adults who screened negative for a possible eating disorder had visited their GP once or twice in the last year, and 36% had visited three or more times. Among adults with a possible eating disorder, 32% had visited once or twice and half (50%) had visited three or more times. The proportion visiting three or more times was highest among those who reported that their feelings about food had a significant negative impact on their lives (56%).

Adults with a possible eating disorder were three times more likely to have seen a GP for both mental and physical problems (18% compared to 6% of those without a possible eating disorder), and more likely to have consulted for a

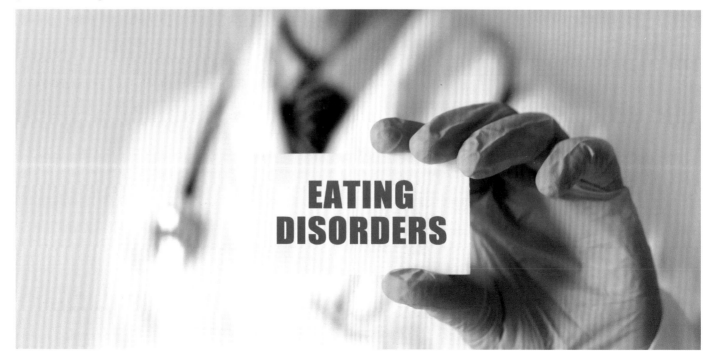

Figure 9: How many times seen a GP in past year, by whether screened positive for a possible eating disorder

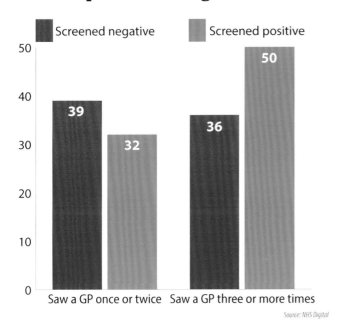

Legend: Screened negative, Screened positive

- Saw a GP once or twice: Screened negative 39, Screened positive 32
- Saw a GP three or more times: Screened negative 36, Screened positive 50

Source: NHS Digital

Figure 11: Whether received any therapy in past year, by whether screened positive for possible eating disorder, experienced significant negative impact

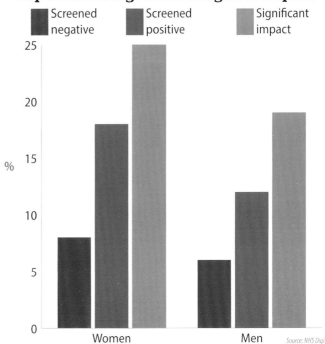

Legend: Screened negative, Screened positive, Significant impact

%

Women / Men

Source: NHS Digital

mental health problem alone (6% and 3% respectively). The proportions who had seen their GP in the last 12 months for a mental health, nervous or emotional problem were highest among those who reported that food had a significant negative impact on their lives: 11% had seen their GP for a mental health, nervous or emotional problem only, and 24% had seen their GP for this and a physical problem as well.

Counselling or therapy for a mental health problem in last year, by whether screened positive for a possible eating disorder

Participants were asked about their use of a range of services. These included current use of psychotherapy, counselling, cognitive behavioural therapy and mindfulness therapy over the past year.

Figure 10: Reasons for GP visits in past year, by whether screened positive for possible eating disorder and experienced significant negative impact

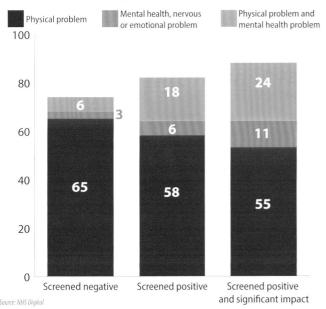

Legend: Physical problem; Mental health, nervous or emotional problem; Physical problem and mental health problem

- Screened negative: 65, 3, 6
- Screened positive: 58, 6, 18
- Screened positive and significant impact: 55, 11, 24

Source: NHS Digital

Adults with a possible eating disorder were more likely than those screening negative to be in receipt of counselling or therapy in the last year (16%, compared with 7% of adults who screened negative). Among adults who screened positive, women were more likely than men to be receiving some type of therapy (18% of women compared to 12% of men). But four in five adults (84%) who screened positive for a possible eating disorder were not receiving such counselling or therapy.

Adults with a possible eating disorder who reported that it had a significant negative impact on their lives were most likely to be in receipt of counselling or therapy; 23% reported this.

The type of therapy most frequently used was counselling, accessed by 7% of all those with a possible eating disorder and 10% of those for whom food had a significant impact on their lives, compared with 2% of other adults without an eating disorder. People with possible eating disorders were also likely to use cognitive behavioural therapy (4% of those for whom food had a significant impact, 5% of all those with a likely eating disorder); psychotherapy or psychoanalysis (5% and 3% respectively); and mindfulness therapy (5% and 3% respectively).

15 December 2020

Sharp rise in number of children in England seeking help for eating disorders

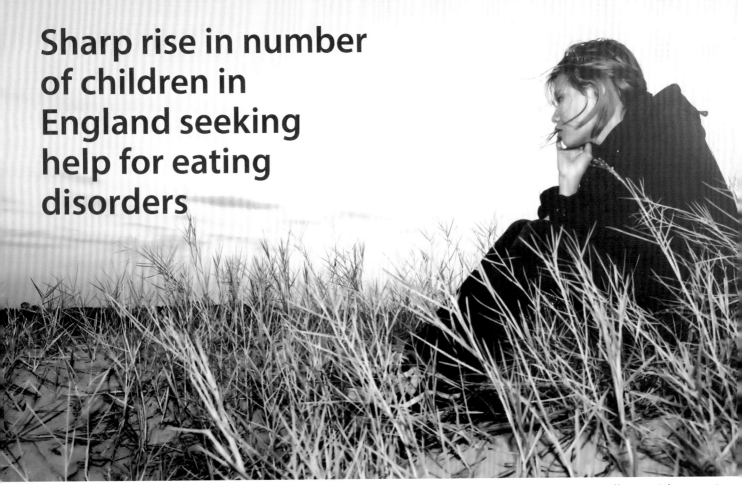

Covid means more young people struggling to access help, as expert warns illness 'thrives in isolation'.

By Sarah Marsh

A doubling of urgent referrals for children with eating disorders combined with a squeeze on services caused by the pandemic has led to an increase in waiting times, with some patients sent hundreds of miles to obtain help, psychiatrists have said.

A staggering one in five women in England may have an eating disorder, according to the NHS Health Survey for England. The figures for 2019 are far higher than those in a comparable survey in 2007.

The number of young people seeking emergency support in the community for anorexia and bulimia reached an all-time high, as mental health practitioners say eating disorders thrive in the isolation brought on by coronavirus. However, available treatment has been further reduced, as most day services are either closed or run with hugely reduced numbers. A leading psychiatrist said the situation was leading to avoidable deaths.

Emergency cases, where people are so unwell they require immediate help, have risen as people are struggling to get timely support, leading to their condition worsening.

A Guardian investigation has found:

♦ The number of urgent referrals for children and young people starting treatment in the community has reached an all-time high of 625, up from 328 at the start of the year and 325 in the same quarter last year, NHS England data shows.

♦ The number of routine referrals starting treatment in the community rose from 915 in April to June 2016 to 1,850 in the first three months of 2020. After the pandemic began, the number of routine referrals starting treatment fell to 1,347. It then rose to a record high of 2,001 in July to September 2020, 38% higher than the previous few months.

♦ In the south of England – including Oxfordshire, Buckinghamshire, Wiltshire and Berkshire – the number of referrals for inpatient care among all ages has shot up by 20% since the pandemic. Approximately 70% of referrals were urgent or emergencies – urgency was determined by the risk to the patient's health and safety. Among this cohort, 20% of referrals were below a BMI of 13, an indicator of potentially life-threatening malnutrition, and 40% had extreme malnutrition requiring urgent treatment.

♦ Waiting times for inpatient mental health admissions for all ages have doubled from 33 to 67 days in the south of the country, with huge individual variations around England.

♦ Separate Guardian research through freedom of information requests found that NHS England spent £10 million over three years sending patients from England to Scotland for treatment, as experts say coronavirus has made the situation worse, expressing concern that out-of-area placements hamper recovery. In the year 2019-

2020, 32 adult patients were forced to travel out of the country for help.

Agnes Ayton, the chair of the Eating Disorder Faculty at the Royal College of Psychiatrists, said there were many reasons behind rising demand, but that 'eating disorders thrive in isolation' and 'people have less social support'. She added that those experiencing problems were less likely to seek help or see a doctor face-to-face due to Covid-19 infection risk.

She said the pandemic had reduced inpatient capacity due to multiple factors, including outdated estates and facilities, infection control measures and staffing levels. 'The pandemic has made things worse because of the closure of day services up and down the country, and the reduction in face-to-face contact for those who have eating disorders means they get worse in isolation,' she said.

She added that patients in the south of England – where she works – were routinely sent to Scotland, mainly to the Priory in Glasgow, which she said 'now have the majority of patients from England.'

'It clearly should not happen and we have been campaigning for years to stop out-of-area placements. These placements are well demonstrated that they cause distress to patients and families because there is limited contact; it has a negative impact on patient outcomes,' she said.

A letter has been written to MPs in Oxfordshire, Buckinghamshire and Wiltshire warning that services are at breaking point. It says: 'This was already an issue before the pandemic hit; the current pandemic has, however, exacerbated the situation with increasing acuity and even higher referral rates.'

Cotswold House, a tertiary referral centre for adult eating disorder care covering the three counties, has been forced due to a lack of resources to accept referrals only for severe anorexia or bulimia.

Ayton said clinicians were reporting an increase in eating disorder referrals in children and adults, and increasing need for hospital admission with growing waiting times for admissions 'even among patients with life-threatening malnutrition'.

She said NHS England had come up with commissioning guidance around what community services should look like, but that there was 'no money attached to it'. As a result, clinical commissioning groups say the guidelines are too expensive to execute, asking local practitioners to be innovative.

'I am beside myself as that is a major risk that the guidelines are either ignored or watered down so that the quality of services will not be improved. I am worried about that,' she said.

'We need research on improving treatment but we cannot even offer timely access to evidence-based treatment and that is a massive problem … I am worried that with Covid-19 and Brexit we will be at bottom of the queue [for funding]. People are dying from eating disorders and these deaths are preventable.'

Claire Murdoch, NHS England's mental health director, said: 'The pandemic has turned lives upside down and hit young people particularly hard, so while a record-high number of young people are in fact getting care for eating disorders, it is sadly a likely fact of the pandemic's impact that more young people will need to seek out support for mental ill-health, which is why the NHS continues to offer face-to-face appointments and inpatient care when needed, while providing the option of phone and video consultations and online support where appropriate.

'Psychiatrists and mental health teams are working to ensure patients get the right care, at the right time and as close to home as possible. Young people who are struggling with an eating disorder also stand to benefit significantly from recently announced rapid access to specialist NHS treatment across England, which will provide access to early intervention, treatment and support.'

16 December 2020

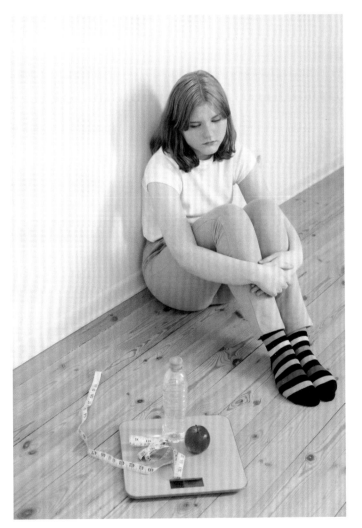

'Deadly illness is thriving': Demand for leading eating disorder charity triples in pandemic with record high

Exclusive: 'A lot of families are contacting us saying my child has deteriorated in six weeks. It is really terrifying for them,' says specialist psychotherapist.

By Maya Oppenheim, Women's Correspondent

Demand for the UK's leading eating disorder charity has tripled during the pandemic with the service experiencing record levels of people coming forward to seek help.

Data shared exclusively with *The Independent* shows overall helpline demand soared by 173 per cent in around a year - rising from 4,277 contacts in February 2020 to 11,686 contacts in January this year.

Beat, the charity which runs the helpline, said they have seen a consistent rise since the Covid crisis hit as they warned lockdown measures could be driving the rise.

Overall helpline demand includes calls, online chats, emails, messages via social media and online support group attendance - with the service used by people suffering from eating disorders, anxious loved ones looking after them, and healthcare workers, teachers or social workers who have concerns they have encountered someone with an eating disorder.

Jess Griffiths, the charity's clinical lead, said: 'A lot of families are contacting us saying my child has deteriorated in six weeks. It is really terrifying for them.

'We are constantly surprised how many people have got in touch with us. Eating disorders tend to come from feeling out of control, and in a pandemic, we are feeling more out of control than ever.

'Then there's also more focus on food and fitness than before. One of the only things we can do on a daily basis is our daily exercise so it has become our focus. Also family are home together more so I think people are more aware of what others are eating.'

Dr Griffiths, a psychotherapist who has specialised in eating disorders for 16 years, said she has worked with young people who may miss their breakfast and lunch, but then eat dinner with their family, but this is more obvious in the wake of lockdown.

'Then there is the issue of panic buying and issues with scarcity,' she added. 'People with eating disorders have rigid ideas on what they think is good or bad food and tend to stick with safe foods. So imagine if this safe food is rice and this has gone in the supermarket.'

Dr Griffiths, who previously had an eating disorder herself but is now fully recovered, said food shortages can also be difficult for people with eating disorders as they may have a meal plan from their dietician or therapist to stick to.

Meanwhile, lockdown measures can make it highly tricky for those with eating disorders due to 'people being more on edge due to being cooped up indoors', she added. On the contrary, she said people who live alone may be struggling as they are isolated and have not had enough support.

'People with eating disorders are very sensitive people,' Dr Griffiths added. 'If you come in with a hard approach, this can make it worse. But as a parent, there is an innate desire to feed your child. So then to see your child rejecting food is very hard.'

She explained while it can be difficult for loved ones to relate to those with eating disorders and they can instead be left feeling frustrated, it is important to recognise there is a range of 'underlying issues which inform' eating disorders.

It is estimated that 1.25 million people in the UK have an eating disorder — such as bulimia and anorexia nervosa — with the majority of those being female. The figure also includes those who binge eat, which can lead to being overweight.

Dr Agnes Ayton, chair of the Eating Disorders faculty at the Royal College of Psychiatrists, told *The Independent*: 'This deadly illness is thriving because many people have lost their support networks alongside access to community services as a result of Covid-19.

'Infection control and social distancing in inpatient units has also led to a reduced number of beds so desperately ill patients are struggling to get help. The government and the NHS must take immediate action to tackle this crisis.'

She called for all medical professionals to have better training in noticing eating disorders early and for services to be 'properly resourced' so patients who manage to get a referral do not have to endure such a lengthy wait for treatment.

NHS England must provide waiting time targets for adults or the 'cruel postcode lottery' for treatment will persist, Dr Ayton said.

The fresh data comes after a report shared exclusively with *The Independent* found eight in 10 women suffering from eating disorders are fearful for their own safety during the second national lockdown which took place in November.

Altum Health, a London-based practice of psychologists, said there had been a surge in people with eating disorders ringing for support after the Covid-19 lockdown.

5 February 2021

Tackling the stigma of eating disorders in men and boys

By Alison Bloomer

The actor Chris Eccleston made the headlines last month when he admitted that he has battled with anorexia for decades and at one point considered suicide.

In his new book, *I Love the Bones of You*, the actor described himself as a 'lifelong body-hater', saying he was 'very ill' with the condition while filming *Doctor Who*. He said he never revealed his struggle before because it's not what working class northern males do.

At the time, a spokesperson for the eating disorder charity Beat said it took courage to speak about having anorexia. 'Doing so helps to combat the stigma and misunderstanding that exists around these serious mental illnesses, especially for men and boys,' they said.

Often seen as a 'female problem', eating disorders in men are frequently under reported, but recent research shows that disordered eating practices may, for the first time, be increasing at a faster rate in males than in females.[1]

In addition, studies suggest that risk of mortality for males with eating disorders is higher than it is for females so early intervention is critical.[2]

Body image is believed to be a big factor. One study found that roughly 90% of teenage boys exercise with the purpose of bulking up.[3] Psychological, genetic, and family influences can also play a role.[2]

Eating disorders - such as anorexia nervosa, bulimia nervosa and binge eating disorder - affect an estimated 1.6 million people in the UK, though the true figure may be higher as many people do not seek help.

Lack of understanding of eating disorders among doctors

Despite the scale of the problem, resources to treat eating disorders are scarce. There are very few specialised treatment centres. People affected are often young and vulnerable, and may avoid detection. However, the earlier a disorder can be diagnosed, the better the likely outcome for the patient.

A recent report from the Public Administration and Constitutional Affairs Committee on the care of people with eating disorders found that there is a lack of understanding of eating disorders among doctors resulting in avoidable deaths.

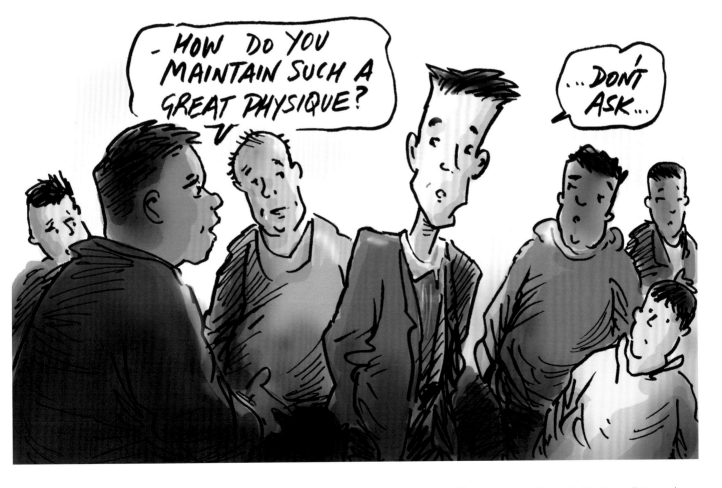

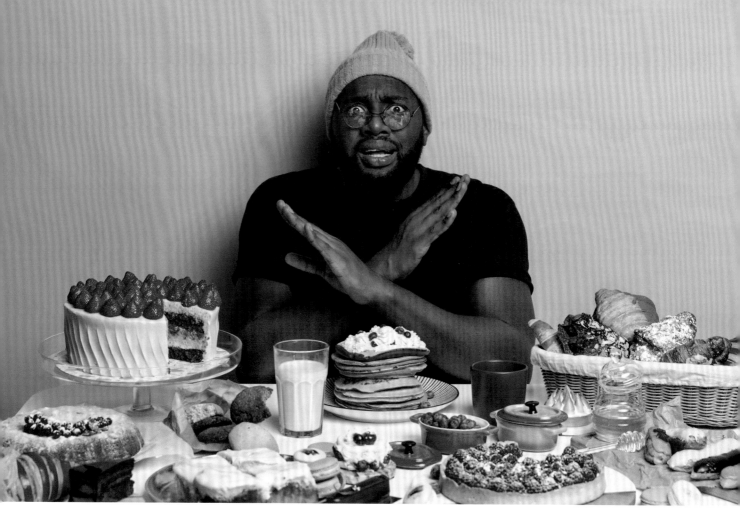

It found that medical staff and GPs, in particular, need significantly more training on the nature of anorexia nervosa and the behaviours that sufferers may display. The report also identifies a series of failings from the NHS to act on recommendations for improving care for patients with eating disorders to avoid unnecessary deaths.

Can GPs intervene earlier in eating disorders?

A study in the British Journal of Psychiatry by the Royal College of Psychiatrists looked at early warning signs of a possible eating disorder in general practice.

The research team, from Swansea University Medical School, examined anonymised electronic health records from GPs and hospital admissions in Wales. 15,558 people in Wales were diagnosed as having eating disorders between 1990 and 2017.

In the two years before their diagnosis, data shows that these 15,558 people had:

♦ Higher levels of other mental disorders such as personality or alcohol disorders and depression

♦ Higher levels of accidents, injuries and self-harm

♦ Higher rate of prescription for central nervous system drugs such as antipsychotics and antidepressants

♦ Higher rate of prescriptions for gastrointestinal drugs (eg. for constipation and upset stomach) and for dietetic supplements (eg. multivitamins, iron).

Therefore, looking out for one or a combination of these factors can help GPs identify eating disorders early.

Dr Jacinta Tan, associate professor of psychiatry at Swansea University and the Welsh representative of the Eating Disorder Faculty in the Royal College of Psychiatrists, said: 'I cannot emphasise enough the importance of detection and early intervention for eating disorders. Delays in receiving diagnosis and treatment are sadly common and also associated with poorer outcomes and great suffering.

'The increased prescriptions by GPs both before and after diagnosis indicates that these patients, even if not known to specialist services, have significantly more difficulties or are struggling. This underlines the clinical need for earlier intervention for these patients and the need to support GPs in their important role in this.'

1. Mitchison D, et al. The epidemiology of eating disorders: genetic, environmental, and societal factors. Clin Epidemiol. 2014; 6: 89–97

2. https://www.nationaleatingdisorders.org/learn/general-information/research-on-males

3. https://www.ncbi.nlm.nih.gov/pmc/articles/PMC3507247/

19 November 2019

www.bjfm.co.uk

Busting myths about eating disorders

Content warning: This blog covers the topic of eating disorders, which can be difficult to read about or discuss. There are no numbers, specifics or eating disorders behaviours included.

By Alice Dalrymple

I have now re-started this blog post 3 times because although I am perfectly happy sharing my day to day struggles with an Eating Disorder with strangers on the internet, putting it out there where people actually know me, feels really scary.

Like many mental health conditions, Eating Disorders can thrive off shame, secrecy, and personal stigma, and it was shame that kept me silent when I was struggling the most. So, it's time to speak up.

An Eating Disorder is a mental health condition where you use the control of food to cope with feelings and other situations. Unhealthy eating behaviours may include eating too much or too little or worrying about your weight or body shape.

Some examples of eating disorders include avoidant/restrictive food intake disorder, bulimia, binge eating disorder, and anorexia. There's no single cause and people might not have all symptoms for any one eating disorder. It's also possible for someone's symptoms, and therefore their diagnosis, to change over time.

I want to start by exploring some common misconceptions when it comes to Eating Disorders.

Myth 1: Someone must be underweight to have an eating disorder

FACT: Often when people think of someone with an Eating Disorder, they think of someone who is significantly underweight. However, although weight loss is typical in anorexia, most people with an eating disorder stay at an apparently "healthy" weight or are "overweight" (as commonly measured by the BMI scale).

If the person does need to restore their weight, this is only one aspect of treatment, and being weight restored does not mean that the person is recovered. The thoughts and behaviours that come alongside the eating disorder also need to be addressed.

Myth 2: Eating disorders are a choice

FACT: Eating disorders are complex illnesses – there is no single cause. Instead they are thought to be caused by a combination of biological, psychological, and sociocultural factors. Eating disorders are extremely distressing for both the individual and their loved ones, and often are accompanied by feelings of shame. They require specialist treatment, but people can and do get better. Eating disorders are mental health disorders and are never a personal choice.

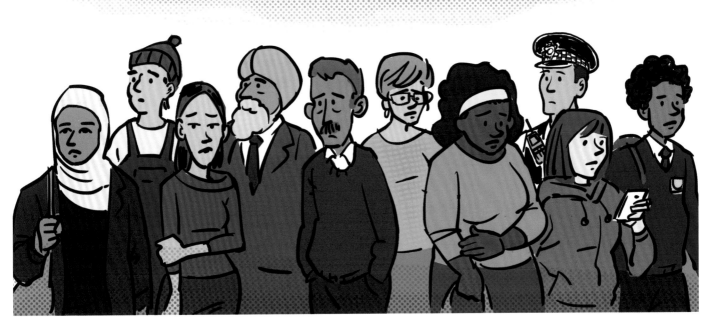

'Eating disorders... ...that only affects young white girls, right?'

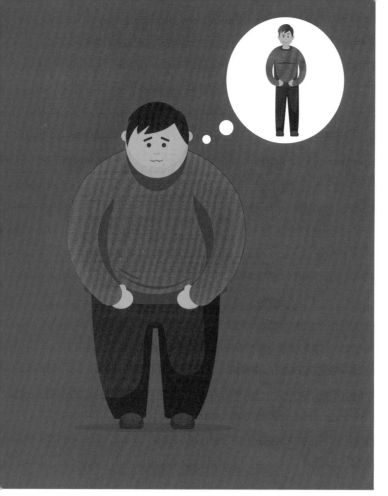

Myth 3: Eating disorders only happen to young girls

FACT: Research shows that eating disorders do not discriminate – they affect people of all genders, ages, ethnicities, sexual orientations, weights, and socioeconomic statuses. Many people think of Eating Disorders as a 'heterosexual, white, female' problem and as a result, males, people of colour and those from the LGBTQ community are less likely to be diagnosed and face greater barriers to treatment.

Myth 4: Eating disorders are a diet gone wrong

FACT: Although for some people, one trigger for an eating disorder may be that they have been dieting, eating disorders are not "a diet that has gone wrong". They are serious mental health disorders which can go on to have adverse effects on physical health which can be fatal.

How these myths affect us

Now we've busted some myths, it's time to get to the scary part. I'm Alice, an Events Manager for Creative Youth Network and I have an Eating Disorder. I have had an Eating Disorder since my teens and it is something which I will continue to be in recovery from for the rest of my life.

I say that because every day I have to make the decision to choose recovery and some days it is easier than others. My Eating Disorder stemmed from control (see Myth #4 – NOT a diet gone wrong) and even now, when I feel overwhelmed, controlling the way I eat or exercise is an easy way for me to feel on top of things. This works, momentarily but then it can lead me to a place which is difficult to climb out of.

Accessibility to Eating Disorder treatment has historically been restricted to people who fit a certain appearance (young, thin, white, female – see Myth #3 for why this is wrong), and in my case this meant when I reached out for help, I was seen as not yet thin enough to need help. The message I heard loud and clear was 'If you want us to help you then you need to lose more weight' and that's exactly what I did, at the further detriment of my physical and mental health, personal relationships and general life.

After time and further requests for help I was able to access the support I needed and I sit today in a much better place when it comes to my body and food. Thankfully, a shift has started to happen to see Eating Disorders as a mental illness with the possible side effect of losing weight, but, there is still a long way to go, especially in understanding the disproportionately unfair access to services for marginalised people.

Eating Disorders do not discriminate, so why do our measurement and treatment systems?

Body image & Eating Disorders

Another reason for sharing my experience is in the relevance of the link between body image and Eating Disorders and the effect it has on our work as a youth support organisation. Talking to colleagues who work in the youth work teams, body image is a recurring theme in many referrals. I'm sadly not surprised as the thin ideal is consistently sold as the key to happiness and health.

Interestingly, when I was my thinnest I was the most unhealthy (and certainly the saddest) I have been in my life but no-one said a thing… apart from to praise me for losing weight. With the rise of social media filters and Instagram nutritionists selling their latest 'Wellness plans' there is no wonder that more and more of us want to change the way that we look.

Contributing to this – the representation of fat people in TV and film, often only awarded the storyline of desperately trying to lose weight or to serve as the butt of everyone's jokes. Judging people for their weight seems to be the last acceptable form of prejudice and I hope within my lifetime that we see a change in this narrative.

There needs to be education around health being a whole spectrum of things and not about making ourselves smaller. This includes considering language we use about bodies and food, especially around those which we have influence (e.g. young people).

I dream of the day that we all celebrate the food that we eat and the amazing things that our bodies do for us.

www.creativeyouthnetwork.org.uk

What is Orthorexia?

Orthorexia has gained increasing attention in the press in recent years, but what is it? Sometimes described as orthorexia nervosa, it describes those who may be seen as having 'unhealthy obsessions' with otherwise healthy eating. Orthorexia usually starts out as a harmless attempt to follow certain healthy eating rules. However, in some cases, these rules start to become all consuming obsessions. At this point, a person may be referred to as having 'orthorexia'. 'Healthy' dietary rules will be followed to an extreme, and the person will become fixated on food quality and purity. Deviations or 'slip ups' from these rigid food rules become highly distressing, and are often taken as evidence that the person is a failure, or has no will power. 'Punishment' is often used following any deviation from these very rigid rules, and may include fasting, increased dietary restriction or strict exercise. Self-esteem becomes wrapped up in sticking to very rigid food rules, and food choices are often thought to be 'superior' to those of others.

Is orthorexia an eating disorder?

Orthorexia is a term coined by Steven Bratman, MD to describe his own experience with food and eating. It is not an officially recognised disorder in the DSM-V, but is similar to other eating disorders – those with anorexia nervosa or bulimia nervosa obsess about calories and weight while someone with orthorexia will obsess about healthy eating (not necessarily about being 'thin' or losing weight). Orthorexia appears to be motivated by health, but there are often additional underlying motivations, which can include safety from poor health, compulsion for complete control, escape from fears, wanting to be thin, improving self-esteem, searching for spirituality through food, and using food to create an identity. These underlying causes are very similar to many of the factors that cause or maintain other known eating disorders.

Why is orthorexia unhealthy?

When food choices become so restrictive, in both variety and calories, health suffers. The diet of someone with orthorexia, despite being designed to provide optimal 'health', is actually likely to be unhealthy, with nutritional deficits specific to the diet they have imposed upon themselves. These nutritional deficits may not always be apparent as a person may continue to 'feel' healthy.

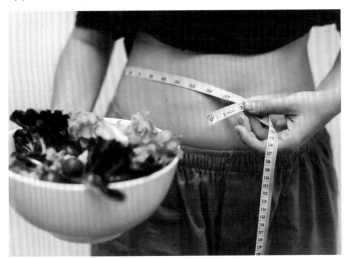

Social problems are often more apparent. A person with orthorexia can easily become socially isolated, often because they plan their life around food. They may have little room in life for anything other than thinking about and planning food intake. Orthorexics lose the ability to eat intuitively – to know when they are hungry, how much they need, and when they are full. Instead of eating naturally they are destined to keep 'falling off the wagon,' resulting in a feeling of failure familiar to followers of any diet. In the long term, obsessions with healthy eating will start to crowd out other activities and interests, impair relationships, and become physically dangerous.

What does recovery from orthorexia look like?

Recovered orthorexics will still eat healthily, but they will achieve a different understanding of what healthy eating is. They will realize that food will not make them a better person and that basing their self-esteem on the quality of their diet is irrational. Their identity will shift from 'the person who eats health food' to a broader definition of who they are – a person who loves, who works, who is fun. They will find that while food is important, it is one small aspect of life, and that often other things are more important.

Do I have orthorexia?

Consider the following questions:

♦ Do you ever wish you could spend less time on food and more time living or doing things you enjoy?

♦ Do you wish that occasionally you could just eat and not worry about food quality?

♦ Does you find it very difficult or anxiety provoking to eat a meal that has been prepared by someone else and not to try to control what is served?

♦ Are you constantly looking for ways foods are unhealthy for you?

♦ Do you spend a lot of time thinking about food or planning what you can and can't eat?

♦ Do you feel guilt or self-loathing when you stray from your diet?

♦ Do you feel in control when you stick to the 'correct' diet?

♦ Have you put yourself on a nutritional pedestal and wonder how others can possibly eat the foods they eat?

The more questions you responded 'yes' to, the more likely it is that you may be suffering from orthorexia, and may need professional support to overcome the rigid obsessional rules associated with this disorder.

11 May 2020

The physical effects of...

Anorexia

Anorexia (anorexia nervosa) has very serious physical effects and complications, as well as a devastating impact upon psychological well being.

The effects of anorexia are both short and long-term. There are the immediate physical effects as the body struggles to function without the nutrients and fuel that it needs. The sufferer is also at risk of developing long-term and potentially life-threatening health problems, particularly if the condition is untreated for many years.

Immediate physical signs of anorexia

Food deprivation has a range of physical effects as the body struggles to cope with insufficient nutrients and calories.

Anorexia sufferers can suffer some or all of the following:

◆ constipation

◆ dizzy spells and faintness

◆ abdominal pains

◆ muscle weakness

◆ poor circulation resulting in feeling constantly cold

◆ dry, yellow coloured skin

◆ early morning waking

◆ bloating

◆ people with anorexia often develop long, fine downy hair on face and body

◆ disrupted menstrual cycles or no periods at all

Anorexia and osteoporosis

Osteoporosis, or 'soft bones', is a disease which results in the density of the bones reducing. This leaves sufferers prone to painful fractures, particularly in the spine and hip, persistent and disabling pain and loss of height.

People with eating disorders are at risk of developing osteoporosis because their bodies are deprived of the vital nutrients bones need in order to grow and remain strong. Calcium is the most important nutrient for the bones.

The risk of osteoporosis is particularly serious for people with eating disorders because dangerous eating patterns commonly develop from the age of 13 and throughout the teens, when the bones are still growing and reaching peak strength.

Anorexia and fertility

Infertility is a serious and common complication of anorexia. If a woman's body fat falls dramatically, she will no longer produce the hormone oestrogen, which is necessary to stimulate ovulation.

Nine out of ten women with anorexia will stop having periods. If the menstrual cycles and ovulation are suppressed for a very long time, this can affect fertility. A recent study found one in five women at an IVF clinic were experiencing problems due to an eating disorder.

The stopping of periods can be permanent, if a sufferer has had untreated anorexia for a long time. But for most women, menstruation will start again once they begin to gain weight. Approximately 80 per cent of women who recover from anorexia will regain their ability to conceive.

If a woman with anorexia does conceive, she faces a high risk of miscarriage and having a low birth weight baby. Any woman who is struggling with an eating disorder should delay pregnancy until she has recovered.

Anorexia and heart problems

Anorexia has the highest mortality rate of all forms of mental illness, with rates of between 10 and 15 per cent. A significant proportion of these deaths are due to heart failure as a result of long-term, severe anorexia.

When anorexia has become this severe, the heart is often damaged. There not enough body fat to protect the heart, anaemia, which weakens the blood, can develop and there is commonly poor circulation. This means that the heart is not able to pump and circulate blood effectively.

Severe anorexia results in the loss of muscle mass, including heart muscle. Consequently, the muscles of the heart can physically weaken, there can be an overall drop in blood pressure and pulse and it can contribute to slower breathing rates.

Studies have shown that the majority of people with anorexia who are admitted to hospital have low heart rates. Common heart problems include arrhythmias (fast, slow or irregular heart beat), bradycardia (slow heart beat) and hypotension (low blood pressure).

Anorexia and neurological (brain) problems

People with severe anorexia may suffer nerve damage that affects the brain and other parts of the body. This can lead to nerve affected conditions including the development of seizures, confused thinking and extreme irritability and numbness or odd nerve sensations in the hands or feet (peripheral neuropathy).

Brain scans show that parts of the brain can undergo structural changes and abnormal activity during anorexic states. Some of these changes return to normal after weight gain, but there is evidence that some damage may be permanent.

Anorexia and anaemia (or blood problems)

Anaemia is a common result of anorexia and starvation. In one study, 38 per cent of anorexic participants had anemia. A particularly serious blood problem is pernicious anaemia, which can be caused by severely low levels of vitamin B12. If anorexia becomes extreme, the bone marrow dramatically reduces its production of blood cells, a life-threatening

Bulimia

Bulimia is an eating disorder with physical effects on the body which are serious, harmful and, left untreated, can result in long-term problems. Although the physical effects of anorexia nervosa, including the condition's mortality rate, are perhaps better recognised, the physical effects of bulimia are multiple and should not be under-estimated. Bulimia effects can, for some, become life-threatening and certainly for many, bulimia can have a long-term health impact.

There are multiple effects from the cycle of binging and purging that is characteristic of bulimia. Bulimia treatment is essential: the longer the condition persists without effective treatment, physical effects become increasingly serious and lasting.

Here, we will break down this

♦ Immediate physical signs of bulimia

♦ Long-term physical effects of bulimia

♦ Treatment and support

Immediate physical signs of bulimia

There are a range of immediate physical effects of bulimia. The effect on each individual will vary according to the pattern of their eating disorder and individual physiology. Physical signs can include:

♦ Russell's sign

♦ Swollen face

♦ Tooth decay

♦ Sore throat

♦ Dehydration

One of the most well-known bulimia effects is 'Russell's sign': calluses on the knuckles and hands caused when inducing vomiting, as in doing so, this part of the hand scrapes against the teeth. Russell's sign, however, is not present in all people with bulimia; many will purge without causing this bulimia effect and may depend on other types of purging (laxatives, over-exercising).

Tooth decay is closely linked to the binge vomit cycle because the contents of the stomach are highly acidic and repeated cycles of vomiting cause tooth enamel to break down through this acidic content. Bad breath is another bulimia effect.

Face swelling is one of the bulimia effects sufferers find most distressing: sometimes described as 'bulimia face', the swelling can make people feel their face 'looks fat'. What is taking place is the body's reaction to self-induced vomiting and the dehydration it causes. The body reacts by trying to hold on to as much water as possible and this is most evident in the parotid glands (around the jawline and side of the face).

Long-term physical effects of bulimia

Bulimia has a devastating impact upon the whole body in the long term, causing multiple serious effects:

♦ Electrolyte imbalance, particularly potassium

♦ Chronic fatigue

♦ Loss or disruption of menstrual cycle

♦ Bone weakness

Electrolytes are electrically charged salts, or ions, used by the body to regulate hydration, together with nerve and muscle function. They are determined by hydration: how much water is present in the body.

A long-term pattern of purging leaves the body's electrolytes in a persistent imbalance, with the risk of effects on heart and kidney function. Potassium is an electrolyte (and also classified as a mineral) which is often depleted by the binge purge cycle and is particularly important for heart function. People with bulimia should have a test of potassium levels and receive a supplement, if required, because very low potassium levels can cause irregular heart rhythms and the breakdown of heart tissue fibres.

Other long-term physical effects of bulimia nervosa and potential risks include menstrual cycle disruption and associated fertility problems. Chronic fatigue caused by the constant depletion of nutrients during purges is also a risk, together with future problems with bone health, due to loss of calcium. Tooth decay caused by bulimia may be permanent and difficult to treat.

Treatment and support

Fortunately, there is good, established bulimia treatment, with strong evidence for its effectiveness. Bulimia treatment is based on a CBT (cognitive behavioural therapy) based approach, supporting individuals to consider the links between their thoughts, feelings and behaviour. It is a practical, problem-solving approach and in bulimia treatment, the triggers for a binge are considered and how this could be overcome by changing the pattern of thoughts, feelings and behaviour.

Treatment is almost always provided in an outpatient setting (seeing a CBT therapist once a week), unless there are other problems which necessitate an inpatient admission. Group support may also be helpful.

Seeking treatment for bulimia as early as possible is very important, both in terms of reducing your risk of long-term, enduring physical side-effects and because it is recognised with bulimia and other eating disorders, early treatment is linked to better outcomes. This is because the longer eating disorders persist, the more entrenched and difficult to treat they become.

Written by clinicians at Schoen Clinic, Newbridge, part of Schoen Clinic UK, which provides specialist mental health services in London, Birmingham and York.

www.newbridge-health.org.uk

'My daughter Nikki Grahame's eating disorder spiralled in lockdown'

The Big Brother star has been battling anorexia since she was a child. Her mother Sue talks about their struggle.

By Eleanor Steafel

When Sue Grahame's daughter was nine, she can remember climbing into her hospital bed at Great Ormond Street and holding her frail little body.

Frightened that Nikki – who had been hospitalised with a bout of anorexia so bad her physician said it was the worst case he'd ever seen – would die, Sue lay beside her daughter and willed her to get better. 'Please get well,' she whispered in her ear. 'I promise you, life is going to be worth living.'

'And it was,' she says. At one point in the Noughties, Nikki Grahame was a household name. The seventh series of Big Brother, in its heyday back in 2006, had made her a reality TV star aged 24. Viewers fell in love with her authenticity and meltdowns, clips of which are still shared on social media today. Back then, reality television was just a bit of fun – a social experiment. In hindsight, what millions loved about Nikki was her fragility.

For her mother and older sister Natalie, watching at home, it was nerve-wracking. Sue always knew, she says, when Nikki 'was going to lose it'.

It wasn't so many years before she got the call inviting her to be a Big Brother housemate that Nikki had been in the throes of the eating disorder which has plagued her since childhood.

From eight to 16, her mother tells me, she spent more time in eating disorder units than at home or in school. That sad statement may soon ring true for many other parents, as eating disorder referrals among young people have doubled during the pandemic, Claire Murdoch, the national mental health director at NHS England, warned this week, with experts blaming a 'loss of control' over their lives.

Anorexia: How to approach someone who you think or know has an eating disorder

Tips from charity Beat

- Get some help for yourself first by talking to a friend or professional about your concerns

- Prepare what you want to say, and how you're going to say it

- Choose a place where you both feel safe and won't be disturbed

- Choose a time when neither of you is angry or upset – avoid any time just before or after meals

- Don't be disheartened if you're met with a negative reaction. Understand that the illness affects how someone thinks and can prevent them from being able to truly believe there is anything wrong with them

- Be aware that they're likely to be feeling guilty, ashamed and very scared

- Be prepared for them to be angry and emotional, or even to say hurtful things

- Don't label them or attempt to trick them into saying they have an eating disorder

- Use 'I' sentences ('I am worried as I've noticed you don't seem happy') instead of 'you' sentences ('you need to get help')

- If they can acknowledge that they have a problem, offer to help them by going to see their GP with them for example

- Have some information about eating disorders to hand – refer to them if the person is able to talk about it, or leave resources behind for them to look at on their own

- If they are not ready to talk about their problem, reassure them that you'll be there when they are. Don't leave it too long before broaching the subject again

- Get young children into treatment. Be persistent and don't give in or wait until they are ready

Indeed, this week, after a gruelling lockdown which saw Nikki's anorexia spiral, she checked herself into a specialist facility for life-saving care, aged 38. Two of her friends set up a GoFundMe page to help raise money for the private treatment she has never been able to afford and so desperately needs.

'She has been battling for most of her life and as you can see, Nikki is now in a very bad way so we need to do something quickly,' they wrote earlier this month.

Speaking via video call from her home in Dorset, Sue, 66, looks exhausted. She has just returned from looking after Nikki at her London flat, ahead of her entering the facility. She weeps as she tells me that this is the worst her daughter has been.

'We've been on this road a long time, 30 years on and off, and I've never seen her this bad,' she sobs. 'I'm frightened that I'll die and she'll have no one to support her. I don't want her to go through any of this alone.'

'While there's breath in my body, and while Nikki is struggling, I don't know how to do anything else other than help her.'

Sue and her ex-husband David first noticed Nikki becoming 'thin and withdrawn' when she was seven. 'One of the girls in her gymnastics team came up to her and said: "Your bum looks big in your leotard." From that moment she started to refuse food.'

At the time, Sue says, theirs 'wasn't a happy house', and she and Nikki's dad went on to divorce. Nikki's relationship with her dad has been 'fiery', she adds, but 'she's always been Daddy's little girl'.

By the time she turned eight, Nikki weighed just under 3st. 'She was a tiny little thing. I was so desperate I can remember actually scooping food with my hand and trying to force it into her mouth.'

In the years that followed, it was the same routine. Nikki would start refusing food, hiding her thinness with baggy clothes, until she would have to be hospitalised. In the units, she would be given a nasogastric tube, or have one sewn into her stomach to help her gain weight, which, Sue says, she would 'just pull out'.

As she got older, the hospital stints became less frequent, though the disease was never far from their lives – as an adult, Nikki has been sectioned more than once following suicide attempts. When the chance for fame came in her twenties, Sue, who was working as a postwoman at the time, was apprehensive but relieved to see her daughter happy.

'Nikki came flying round. She sat on the bed. Her phone rang and they said "We'd like to invite you to be a housemate",' she recalls.

'She was jumping up and down, she was so delighted. I sat there and thought "Oh my God". I'd never seen the show and I thought "is she going to cope?"'

'She said "Mum, it's the best day of my life!"'

For a while, Nikki was a guest on every game show and the star of every producer's next reality TV idea. A second stint in the Big Brother house came in 2010, and a third on Big Brother Canada in 2016. She published two books in 2009 and 2012, detailing her experiences with anorexia. But as the fame fell away, the eating disorder took hold again.

'When you're up there and you're having a great time, working your socks off, it's marvellous. But then it can stop. And Nikki said she did feel quite lost when it stopped,' explains Sue.

Lockdown, she says, was a final blow. Nikki had been working in a school before the pandemic. Having spent so much of her own childhood in hospital, she had recently gone back to education, taking courses in English and Science. She had just completed a course on caring for children with special needs when lockdown began. 'She's been trying to further herself,' she adds.

Covid put a temporary stop to that and Nikki, who lives alone, suffered with 'terminal loneliness', as Sue puts it.

'This last year has just about floored her… From the first lockdown, it was hellish. She struggled because she couldn't go to the gym. Then in December she fell down and cracked her pelvis in two places and broke her wrist. I stayed with her for three or four weeks because she couldn't do anything.'

It was only when Nikki's friends saw her again recently, and realised how thin she had become, that they decided something must be done to help and set up the crowdfunding page. It exceeded the goal of £50,000 in a matter of days, with donations now over £67,000.

Sue is praying this latest bout of treatment – more 'holistic' than at NHS eating disorder units – will help Nikki once and for all.

'I only hope that she will be brave and let the help in. I feel slightly more hopeful because it's not people forcing you to put on weight. It's nurturing as well. She needs a good bit of that right now. She needs to learn to like herself.'

Thirty years ago, Sue held her daughter in her hospital bed, willing her to believe life would be worth staying around for. She is still making her that same promise now. 'I said to her: "It's your 40th next year. Come on, we're going to plan something big. You do have things to look forward to. Let's start again."'

For advice and support on anorexia, contact Beat, the UK's eating disorder charity

25 March 2021

Nikki Grahame: No one should be dying of eating disorders in 2021, says charity calling for more adult support

'Adult eating disorder services are chronically underfunded; waiting time targets are not imposed.'

By Serina Sandhu

People should not be dying of eating disorders in 2021, a charity has said in the wake of the death of reality TV personality Nikki Grahame, who had anorexia for most of her life.

Anorexia and Bulimia Care (ABC) said early intervention and age-appropriate support is key to helping individuals but added that services for adults are 'chronically underfunded'.

Ms Grahame, who was a contestant on Channel 4's *Big Brother* in 2006 and later starred in her own reality show *Princess Nikki*, died on Friday at the age of 38. She had recently received treatment for an eating disorder at a specialist clinic.

Joanne Byrne, chief executive of ABC, described Ms Grahame's death after 'a 30-year struggle' as 'tragic', saying it highlighted 'the need for accessible and ongoing, whole-person treatment for those living with eating disorders, regardless of age'.

An estimated 1.25 million people in the UK are affected by eating disorders.

'Adult eating disorder services are chronically underfunded; waiting time targets are not imposed as they are for eating disorder services for children and adolescents under CAMHS (Child and Adolescent Mental Health Services),' Ms Byrne told *i*.

'Early intervention, and ongoing age-appropriate disorder-specific treatment, is crucial to reducing the duration of illness and improving the chance of a full recovery. Eating disorders are treatable and recovery is possible. No one should be dying of an eating disorder in 2021.'

A 2017 report from the Parliamentary and Health Service Ombudsman on how NHS eating disorder services are failing patients recommended that the Government ensure there is parity between available support for adults and young people.

But Gemma Oaten, the patron and charity manager for Seed Eating Disorder Support Services, who knew Ms Grahame personally, said there is still not enough support services.

'One thing I know that Nikki's death will create is an awareness and, my God, there has been so much more conversation happening because of this… Nikki's death will not be in vain and she will leave a legacy and I believe that legacy will be to save lives,' she said.

Ms Oaten, an actress, said her parents founded Seed 21 years ago because her story was 'very similar to Nikki's'.

'And I am here and I am recovered and I am alive and I want people to remember that there can be hope. There is actually hope.

'The sooner somebody speaks out, the quicker they can get help and support and the sooner we can bring that person back and away from the eating disorder.'

With Ms Grahame's condition worsening during the coronavirus pandemic, her friends set up a fund-raising page to help her access support. It said the basic treatment she had been receiving from the NHS was not working and that her only option was to seek intensive care privately.

At the end of March, her mother, Sue Grahame, told ITV's *This Morning* that her daughter had been affected by the closure of gyms and feelings of loneliness in the pandemic.

She also recounted how her daughter spent time receiving treatment as a child and teenager, adding that parents should try and get help as soon as possible.

The NHS said: 'New and expanding community-based mental health care will provide treatment and support for 370,000 adults – including those with eating disorders – closer to home, and the NHS has committed to increasing investment in mental health services faster than the NHS budget, creating a ring-fenced local investment fund worth at least £2.3 billion a year by 2023/24.'

The Department of Health and Social Care said it is crucial people with an eating disorder get 'the support they need, when they need it'.

'Our Mental Health Recovery Action Plan is backed by £500 million to ensure we have the right support in place over the coming year to help people with a variety of mental health conditions, including eating disorders.'

Anyone living with an eating disorder can contact Anorexia and Bulimia Care or Seed for support

13 April 2021

'I missed out on anorexia treatment because of BMI guidelines, leaving me in worst state I've ever been'

BMI is used to determine treatment for eating disorders, and can be a gatekeeping tool for year-long waiting lists for vital care.

By Jasmine Andersson

Two women who missed out on vital care for eating disorders because of BMI restrictions are calling for the metric to be scrapped for good.

They are backing fresh calls by the Women and Equalities Committee to drop the index as it is a 'dangerous' tool that 'flies in the face of science' and exacerbates issues with body image and weight shaming.

For Cara and Joss, their BMI was used to determine whether they qualified for anorexia treatment. NICE advises using the metric 'with caution', but both women have found it is often relied upon to combat year-long waiting lists.

Cara Lisette, 30, was told she didn't meet the BMI range for treatment when she approached her GP about struggling with a potential relapse at the beginning of 2019. Cara had a history of anorexia, and she was first diagnosed at the age of 13.

By the time she was assessed for care nine months later, she was told she was too ill for therapy because her cognitive function had deteriorated.

'I visited my GP in January, and I was told my BMI was too high for me to get diagnosed with anorexia,' she told i.

'By the time I was given an appointment for care in September, I was moved onto the urgent waiting list. My deterioration was so rapid that then I missed the window to see anybody for weekly therapy and then I had to go to a clinic every day.'

The 30-year-old said having the help she needs judged by her BMI is 'really invalidating.'

'When you're not given that help, you either function with an eating disorder, which isn't a very nice way to live, or you end up just deteriorating like I did,' she added.

Joss Walden, 28, was also denied treatment because her BMI did not meet the criteria. By the time she was admitted to hospital, she was 'in the worst physical and mental state I'd ever been in.'

'Although I had a very low BMI, I was told I couldn't qualify for inpatient treatment and I was left with just GP monitoring,' she told i.

'One evening, my breathing had gone funny. I was actually at a point where I didn't to go to sleep at night because I literally didn't know if I was going to wake up in the morning.

'I was so scared I breached patient-doctor confidentiality and I rang my GP's home phone. I found her number in a directory. When she picked up she was so shocked. I said to her "please, you need to do something."'

'In the end, I had to refer myself to a hospital in London. They asked me for my BMI, which in the adolescent services was the cutoff for when you should get help. This nurse said it was too high, and they couldn't help me.

'A few weeks later I was admitted to an inpatient ward in London at the worst physical and mental state I'd ever been in.'

Joss quit university while she was treated for two years. Now, she has returned to university to study Health Psychology, and she has spent years calling for the BMI criteria to be scrapped.

'I think BMI is playing a massive part in my experience of accessing help, of being acknowledged as someone who maybe needs support, and people don't take you seriously,' she said.

When you meet someone or you have a code spread when you say 'look I'm really struggling with anorexia again,' but if I have a healthy, if not high BMI, it's dismissed, and I'm told 'are you struggling with your mental health? Is it just an anxiety disorder?''

'With cancer, you would never put someone on a year-long waiting list if they were desperately sick. With eating disorders, I can never get my head around why people have to prove that they're that unwell,' she added.

A Department of Health and Social Care spokesperson said: 'With over 6 in 10 adults overweight or living with obesity it is important that we take action to help people live healthier lives, and our approach is guided by the latest research and emerging evidence. NHS England has been clear it does not support the use of BMI thresholds.'

9 April 2021

Children as young as 10 rushed to A&E as eating disorder cases 'go through the roof'

Special report: lockdown has seen more children dangerously ill with eating disorders

By Jonathan Humphries

Children as young as 10 are arriving in hospital dangerously ill as the number of young people suffering with eating disorders goes 'through the roof'.

Alder Hey Children's Hospital's specialist Eating Disorders Service has seen referrals increase by around 23%, and the young patients arriving are sicker.

During the months of the coronavirus pandemic the service has seen the highest level of demand since it began.

A report into the effects of lockdown on eating disorder service at Alder Hey said it had seen: 'An increase in the number of children and young people that are presenting at their first assessment as being at high physical risk'.

The service has also seen 'a decline in the health of young people known to the service that, prior to lockdown, were recovering from an eating disorder and working towards improving both their physical and mental health.'

Sufferers of eating disorders, which include anorexia, bulimia and binge eating disorder, say that their anxiety and difficulties controlling their illness have increased markedly during the three national lockdowns.

And the life threatening severity of the illness was brought into sharp relief last week when former Big Brother star Nikki Grahame died at just 38 after a long battle with anorexia.

One community support group, Talking Eating Disorders Liverpool (TEDS), says it has also seen around a 50% increase in the number of adults and children seeking help.

The ECHO spoke to senior doctors at Alder Hey who described how the effects of lockdown have meant children are arriving at hospital in a far more serious physical condition than before.

Dr Vivienne Crosbie, consultant clinical psychiatrist and clinical lead for Alder Hey's Eating Disorder Service, told the ECHO: 'There's been about an increase of 23% in the number of young people who have been referred or accepted into our service, about a quarter more than we had last year.

'More significantly, what we have seen is that over the last year more young people present to our service when they might already be really quite poorly with an eating disorder.

'They have come quite late, having not been able to access some of the universal services they might have accessed in other times; things like GPs, things like school nurses because they are not in school.

'So this has meant by the time they get to us they might need a period of physical health inpatient care to stabilise them.'

Her colleague, consultant general paediatrician Dr Francine Verhoeff, who specialises in eating disorders, said the lockdowns meant referrals had 'gone through the roof'.

Due to investment in the service over the past 15 years, Dr Verhoeff said doctors in Alder Hey had been catching eating disorders earlier - but since lockdown she has seen far more young patients in alarming physical conditions.

She said: 'When you lack nutrition in your body, your body sort of slowly shuts down. The symptoms we see with children, they are very dizzy, sometimes faint, their heart rate is really low, they feel cold, for girls periods might have stopped.

'The reasons why families often attend A&E is that their child becomes so dizzy, with fainting, that they then and there decide to attend the emergency department - or families become really concerned because they notice a significant weight loss or their son or daughter feels really cold.

'Or they can notice a significant change in the mood of the child so they become isolated, with quite low mood, so they don't go out with their friends any more.

'But with lockdown you might not have noticed that so quickly because nobody was going out.'

Dr Verhoeff said the majority of patients referred to the service are aged around 14 or 15, but the youngest is around 10.

18 April 2021

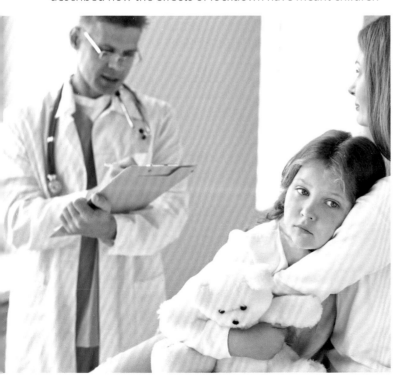

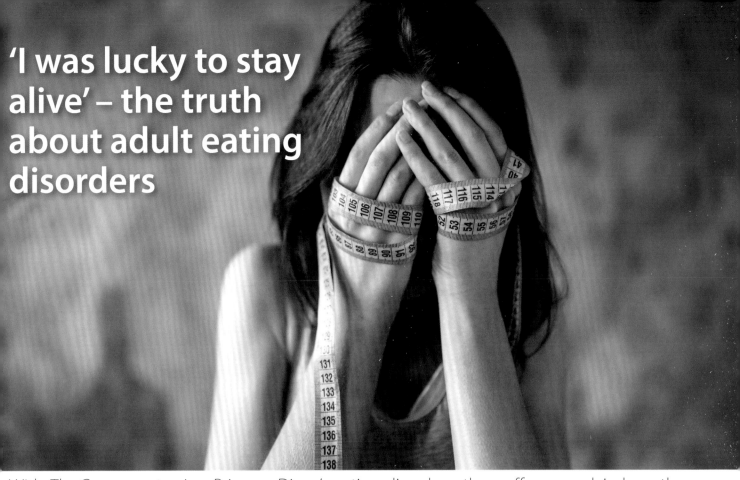

'I was lucky to stay alive' – the truth about adult eating disorders

With *The Crown* portraying Princess Diana's eating disorder, other sufferers explain how they have battled to get treatment.

By Rosa Silverman

When Aimee Yates first began to lose weight, around the age of 30, nobody was too alarmed. Yates had a good job with the NHS and her life seemed to be on track, but she was becoming increasingly anxious as her friends began settling down, having children and buying properties. She was deriving a growing sense of relief from controlling what she ate.

'I felt quite ineffective and couldn't control my life and achieve the things other people were,' she says. 'Though I wasn't consciously wanting to lose weight, I very much didn't want my weight to go up, and my fear of my weight going up led to it going down. Without me realising it, my meals became smaller, my diet more restrictive.'

Before developing anorexia, she had weighed about eight stone. By the time the eating disorder landed her in hospital, she was four-and-a-half stone.

About 1.25 million people in the UK are believed to have an eating disorder, according to the charity Beat. And though we have become far better at discussing mental health problems in recent years, there remains a particular stigma around eating disorders.

The subject is being brought to the fore by the new series of *The Crown*, which was aired this weekend, and depicts graphic scenes of Princess Diana's struggles with bulimia. The Princess of Wales' decision to speak out about her 'secret disease' shed new light on the taboo subject of eating disorders. 'You inflict it upon yourself because your self-esteem is at a low ebb, and you don't think you're worthy or valuable,' she said in her famously candid *Panorama* interview in 1995. It would ease the way for others to speak out and seek help, in what became known as the 'Diana effect'.

Though public perceptions have improved since, the numbers affected by eating disorders continue to rise and the diagnosis still carries a sense of shame and stigma, sometimes born of a misplaced belief that somehow sufferers are 'choosing' disordered eating. This is particularly true when an eating disorder develops in adulthood, as it did in Diana's case.

For Yates, now 46 and living in Cambridge, the age at which she presented with symptoms did affect the way she was treated.

'I went to see a GP and it wasn't a good experience,' she says. "She told me, 'if you were a teenager I'd refer you to the eating disorder service, but you're an adult, so it's your choice to eat or not". I did think, '"I'm old enough to know better, this shouldn't be happening to me".'

As an adult living alone, she was able to conceal what she ate. 'People could see I was still working and functioning well. Friends told me afterwards I was so independent and such a strong woman, they didn't really believe what they were thinking when they saw my weight loss.'

Still, she insisted on being referred to an eating disorder service and was put on a waiting list several months long for outpatient treatment.

'[Meanwhile] my weight continued to slip down,' says Yates. 'I became physically ill. I was so weak... I was staying with my mum and she had to lift a cup to my lips. I was very sleepy, I couldn't do anything for myself.'

At that point she contacted the eating disorder service and was admitted to hospital in London a few days later. 'I was lucky to stay alive for those few days,' she says. She remained in hospital for 10 months, until her heart was stable enough for outpatient treatment.

But she'd 'never fully dealt with the psychological issues', she says. 'So I began binge-eating and for a period suffered from bulimia. I was trying to make myself vomit about 100 times a day.'

Rhiannon Pursall, from Warwick, also knows what it's like to watch yourself slide into disordered eating during adulthood. Now 35, she was in her early 20s and at Sheffield University when it started. 'I'd never had any hang-ups about my body or food,' she says. '[But] I always had that feeling of being not quite sure I was good enough in many areas, and during third year I found myself comparing myself a lot to other girls... There was a sense of comparison and wanting to better myself.'

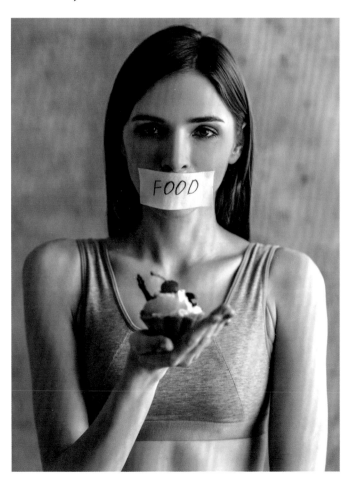

She grew addicted to visiting the gym, where she 'discovered there was this amazing world where you could watch the number of calories you'd burned on the treadmill and translate that into extra calories [to eat] that evening. Then I thought, "if I don't eat more, I'll feel even better tomorrow", and it just spiralled. It was completely out of my control'.

Her illness worsened as the years went on until she went to her GP and was immediately referred to an eating disorder service, but had to wait for treatment. In the meantime, her weight plummeted further – the only clothes that would fit her were children's ones. Services and campaigns are, she says, 'all very much geared to prevention and young people and it's almost like "oh, sorry we missed you".'

Acknowledging that you have an eating disorder can be hard in adulthood, says Dr Bijal Chheda-Varma, a chartered psychologist and cognitive behavioural therapist at Nightingale Hospital. 'It's very shame-based... The key issue is that it's the shame that stops people from coming to clinicians.'

Each time a celebrity shares their own struggles with a mental illness, as Diana did, clinicians do see a slight uptick in those with symptoms coming forward, she says. 'But there is a taboo. The most unfortunate myth is [eating disorders] are... vanity-based, when there's such a range of complexity. I've sometimes heard dads of teenage girls or partners of adult women [saying to them] "What's not to understand? Just eat healthily!"'

In fact, such illnesses are born of a desire to regulate emotions with food; a need for control and a yearning for numbness, she explains.

'The complexity increases with adulthood because we then need to look at what could have triggered it,' she says. 'Adults become high-functioning; they may be holding down jobs and be married with families. Life becomes more complex.'

Treatment, as well as public perception, has improved in the years since Diana spoke out. Where once people were admitted to hospital, often far away from home and for long periods of time, there is now a greater understanding of the value of community treatment instead; of keeping people with their families and social networks.

Yates is a healthy weight today, but still struggles with binge-eating. Pursall is currently recovering.

Experts say the Diana effect endures to this day – and hope the modern retelling of her experiences in *The Crown* will help to improve understanding of eating disorders.

15 November 2020

Fitness influencer opens up on his battle with an eating disorder

'I had no idea what I was doing. I essentially just starved myself and went into phases of literally eating very little food.'

For a lot of men, there is a stigma surrounding eating disorders - much like the way mental health problems are treated.

By Alex Roberts

Eating disorders exist in men - and we know they do - yet you'd be hard pressed to find someone willing to admit they've suffered from one. Finding someone able to speak honestly about their experiences is equally as tricky.

In the male population, disordered eating patterns are a taboo topic too often brushed aside. But the situation in the fitness industry and professional sport is even worse.

Earlier this year, former bodybuilder and fitness model Jamie Alderton told JOE about the dangers of getting 'shredded' for a bodybuilding competition.

He recalled how a fellow competitor used to chew biscuits up and then spit them out again. Alderton himself admitted to buying cakes for his wife, just so he could watch her eat them.

With two million YouTube subscribers, Matt Morsia (a.k.a MattDoesFitness) is one of the biggest fitness influencers on the planet.

He has also battled an eating disorder.

Speaking to JOE in the week before Christmas, Morsia says his background in athletics gave rise to disordered eating patterns.

He said: 'I competed in athletics for almost ten years - I was a long run triple jumper.

'In those events in particular, your body weight is crucial.'

Competing in any sport where you are judged according to your body weight has the potential to wreak havoc on your mental health and subsequent relationship with food.

Those words ring true for Morsia, a former school teacher from Kent.

'If you're trying to jump far, if you're really heavy it's obviously not going to happen. So as long as you can maintain performance, being as light as you possibly can… Well, there's a direct correlation between that and jumping further.'

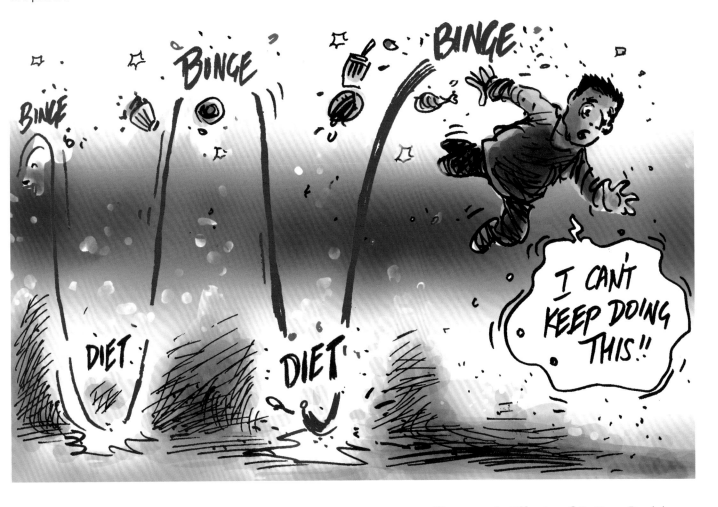

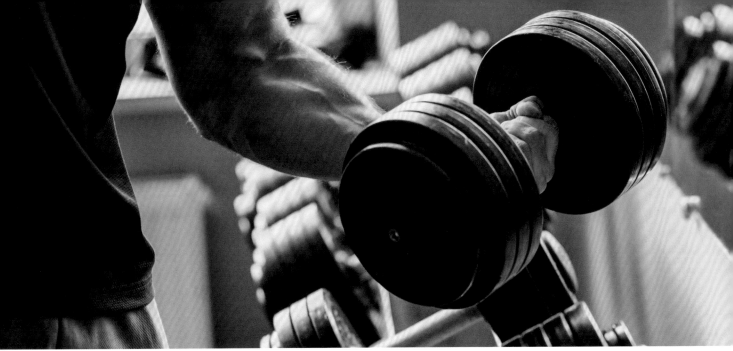

Morsia says these pressures led to disordered eating.

'In that instance, it made sense to lose weight. 'In doing that, because I had no idea what I was doing, I essentially just starved myself and went into phases of literally eating very little food.'

He says his obsessiveness made the problem worse.

'I had no idea about protein, macronutrients or anything like that. I've got quite an all-or-nothing personality, and I think that's quite common in people with disordered eating.

'I was starving myself, and then I'd say "Right, I'll do my competition and then after it, I'll have a cheat day".'

This might sound manageable in theory, but in practice it proved anything but.

'As the summer went on, I'd be competing every weekend for about three months.

'As the season progressed, that starvation got more and more intense.'

Morsia's planned cheat meals soon spiralled out of control.

'What started out as a cheat meal… I'd finish my competition, go out and buy some doughnuts, that then increased to become a cheat day, then it's a cheat weekend.

'Then it just got to the point where I was eating 20,000 calories in the space of 40 hours over that weekend, just literally cramming in as much food. I didn't even want it, I was just cramming in as much food as I physically could, to the point where I'd be throwing up because I'd eaten so much crap.'

He says this is inevitable for anyone on a crash diet.

'If you starve yourself and restrict calories to that extent, it's extremely likely that at some point you're going to rebound, and when you do that you're gonna go nuts and eat uncontrollably.

'I'd be full up, and still be eating random stuff like cream cakes that I didn't even want. It was literally uncontrollable, I couldn't stop myself eating food.'

Matt's eating disorder became a vicious circle of starvation followed by extreme binge eating.

'I'd freak out and make the starvation even more extreme. The more extreme the starvation, the next binge would become more pronounced.'

Morsia is now intent on educating others that weight loss itself isn't necessarily a healthy goal to set. He points to the fact that weight training will increase muscle mass and therefore the number on the scales, but by all barometers, health will have improved immeasurably.

'People tend to go on these extreme, short-term crash diets that generally involve massive calorie restriction. Again, chances are you'll rebound and end up bigger, heavier and fatter than you were before.'

When asked why eating disorders aren't discussed in men as much as they are in women, Morsia said notions of gender stereotypes are probably to blame.

'It's a societal thing, I guess. Historically, men have been told to "man up" and that kind of thing. If you're a guy, I guess admitting you have an eating disorder was seen as embarrassing, and you wouldn't want to admit that.'

Morsia is fine with opening up about his battles, but he understands why the majority of sports people don't.

'I'm happy to talk about it - it's a bit weird, but I don't mind talking about eating disorders.

'I guess if you're a sports person, it's probably easier to justify it because you think there's a reason why you're doing it.'

Self-imposed restrictions are one thing, but sporting bodies arguably need to do more to help.

British Gymnastics have recently faced calls to review the way they train athletes after numerous young stars alleged abuse at the hands of affiliated coaches. Among other issues, coaches have been accused of instilling a culture of belittlement and body shaming - which could exacerbate problems in those prone to disordered eating.

February 2021

Coronavirus pandemic could have long-term effects on people with eating disorders

Researchers looked at data from 129 people recruited online who were experiencing or in recovery from an eating disorder during the early stages of lockdown.

By Paul Gallagher, Health Correspondent

People with eating disorders could be at risk of suffering long-term consequences from the impacts of the coronavirus pandemic, researchers have warned.

The fallout from routines being disrupted in lockdown, a focus on food and exercise which came to dominate the public conversation, and healthcare moving online, could all have lasting effects, academics from Northumbria University in Newcastle said. While positive messaging around diet and fitness can be beneficial to the majority of people, it is important to recognise these can be 'triggering or upsetting' for others, their paper published in the Journal of Eating Disorders said.

The study looked at data from 129 people recruited online who were experiencing or in recovery from an eating disorder during the early stages of lockdown. Participants, who were aged between 16 and 65 and mostly female, were asked about the overall impact of the pandemic on their eating disorder symptoms and almost 90 per cent said they had become worse.

Out of healthy routines

Researchers said they identified key themes including disruption to living situations, increased social isolation and reduced access to usual support networks, changes to physical activity rates and changes to relationship with food. They said one of the major challenges faced by people with an eating disorder was a reduction in healthcare service provision, as well as discrepancies in access to healthcare services.

Erica Matthews, 21, a full-time student from Norfolk who has been recovered for about four years after first recognising she had an eating disorder at the age of 12, told i the pandemic had 'massively' affected her mental health.

She said: 'I used to be able to go out and go for a walk, meet up with friends, go to the library for studying and meet with family for coffee. Once we were put in lockdown, all of that freedom went away and a new routine had to be created.

'Personally I don't think I'll get back to pre-pandemic normal for at least a couple of years. Too much has happened and it's going to take me a while to feel at ease again. The world just feels like a more anxious place than before, and I completely empathise with everyone who is experiencing increased anxiety levels.'

Some participants in the study felt video calls, rather than the usual face-to-face appointments, were having a detrimental effect because seeing themselves on a screen made them more aware and more critical of their appearance. The researchers recommended service providers assess the appropriateness of technologies for providing remote support.

Lack of control

Disruption to routine and perceived control was another issue for many, with one participant saying their lack of control over study, work and socialising had led to them focusing more on control around food. Like much of the population, the majority of people questioned said they had spent more time online in lockdown and 55 per cent said the increase had made their eating disorder symptoms worse. Some felt talk around the general public's fear of gaining weight was 'particularly triggering'.

Researchers said lessons learned from the pandemic could be relevant to other public health emergencies or for future circumstances where there may be periods of lockdown, food shortages or social isolation.

Dr Dawn Branley-Bell, co-author of the paper, said: 'Our findings highlight that we must not underestimate the longevity of the impact of the pandemic. Individuals with experience of eating disorders will likely experience a long-term effect on their symptoms and recovery. It is important that this is recognised by healthcare services, and beyond, in order to offer the necessary resources to support this vulnerable population now and on an on-going basis.'

Beat, a national charity for people with eating disorders, has seen an 81 per cent increase in contact across all Helpline channels. This includes a 125 per cent rise in social media contact and a 115 per cent surge in online group attendance.

Tom Quinn, Beat's Director of External Affairs, said: 'We have seen first-hand the devastating impact the pandemic has had on those suffering from or vulnerable to eating disorders and their loved ones. More and more people are reaching out to our Helpline services, and we are prepared to support anyone in need at this time.'

24 August 2020

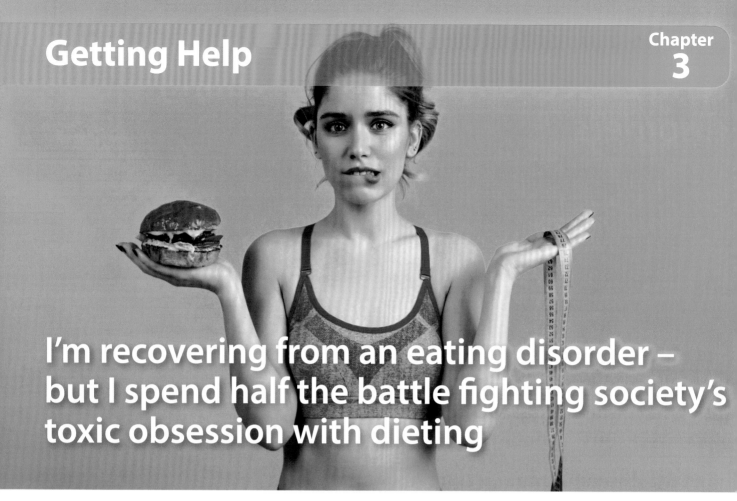

I'm recovering from an eating disorder – but I spend half the battle fighting society's toxic obsession with dieting

I can't buy a sandwich or cook from an online recipe without being confronted with the numbers I want to unlearn. I finally recognise their harm, but the world won't let me forget.

By Tasha Kleeman

Nothing reveals the ubiquity of diet culture so starkly than trying to recover from an eating disorder. Instructed by my dietician to regain a 'normal' pattern of eating, I looked desperately around me for benchmarks. Instead, everywhere I looked, I was confronted with behaviour that I had come to associate with disorder. From my morning newspaper and my Instagram feed, to conversations overheard in supermarkets and among my colleagues and friends, everyone seemed to be worrying about their weight. Looking forward to a return to normality, I instead emerged from hospital to find the signs of my eating disorder writ large on the world.

In my first job back in the 'real world', I found myself, in some dark twist of fate, in an office obsessed with health and fitness. Gym chat was more commonplace than small-talk about the weather, and I couldn't enter the communal kitchen without hearing what new diets people were trying, how many calories were in their M&S 'Balanced for you' ready meals and what horrific gym class they were attending that day to cleanse themselves of the sins of last night's Indian takeaway.

At the desk to my left was a man subsisting entirely on Huel: meal replacement shakes supposedly containing all the nutrients necessary for a perfectly balanced diet (everything but the joy of course – but joy won't get you a six-pack or allow you to work through your lunch break). Others attended gym classes like it was a religion (with all the guilt of a good Catholic), or drank herbal teas promising to eliminate belly fat. While some were unable to eat a piece of cake brought in for someone's birthday without ruminating on how 'naughty' they were for eating it, and what rigorous exercise they would now have to put themselves through to make up for it. In my whole eight months there, I don't think I ever saw anyone eat a sandwich.

I don't mean to seem judgemental. I truly believe that everyone should be left alone to eat whatever makes them happy. However, coming from an environment in which food was so fraught with fear, anxiety and shame, I was surprised and saddened to see so much of that familiar anxiety and control reflected in my new surroundings.

Distancing myself from the calorie-counting that became all-consuming during my illness also proved difficult. Once, as I was checking out of an online food order, Ocado kindly suggested I swap my yoghurt for a lower fat version and save some calories, while Citymapper regularly provides me with an illustrated representation of the food I would burn off if I chose to walk to my destination rather than get the bus. I cannot buy a sandwich from Pret, eat at most chain restaurants or cook from an online recipe without being confronted with the numbers I am trying to unlearn. I finally recognise their tedium and toxicity, but it seems the world won't let me forget.

We live in anxious times. In the war against obesity, meals must come with warnings and colour-coded labels. With environmental pressures mounting, food comes laden with moral and political significance, not to mention large helpings of guilt. Increasingly, we eat not in tune with our bodies but according to externalised rules. As a consequence of my own extreme practice of this, I am still learning how to get back in touch with my hunger and fullness signals. As I look around me at a world obsessed with quantifying food, however, I wonder if this is a problem unique to those recovering from anorexia.

Of course, there is nothing new about this obsessive pursuit of thinness, or the pressure placed on women, in particular, to shrink their bodies and minds to fit into an unrealistic beauty ideal. However, in this age of Instagram, diet culture has been magnified to terrifying proportions. Photoshopping, which used to be a problem of glossy magazines, is now a mass commodity, reflected not just in the booming plastic surgery industry, but available to all with photo filters and apps like Facetune.

Absurd products, like appetite-suppressant lollipops and detox teas, proliferate, and come sponsored by celebrities with enormous followings. A whole new industry has emerged, in which Fitspos and foodies with huge cult followings provide exemplary models of 'healthier' lives. Thanks, in part, to these influencers, our supermarkets profit from a whole new food group. We live in an age of 'courgetti', 'boodles' and sweet potato toast: poor substitutes of the real thing but gloriously carb-free. You can even buy low-calorie ice-cream promising 'guilt-free indulgence' (as if there's something morally incriminating about opting for the real thing).

If that wasn't enough, technology increasingly offers up more opportunities to quantify our health goals: we can track our steps, sleep cycles and heart rates on a FitBit, or track the calories in every mouthful with MyFitnessPal. Diet culture, it seems, has never been so lucrative.

I do not mean to undermine the very real public health challenge posed by rising rates of obesity, nor deny the reality that many of us should be eating more healthily than we do. However, I seriously question many of the measures offered as a solution to these problems. At the day hospital I attended, we would joke that the only people who actually weigh out the advised portion sizes on the front of cereal packets are those with anorexia. From experience, I can attest that 30g of Shreddies is not a nourishing breakfast. In reality, many of the well-meaning public health regulations and messaging around weight loss serve to perpetuate damaged relationships with food, imposing moral judgements onto food and bodies that do more harm than good.

As any seasoned dieter will know, restriction inevitably results in overindulgence and food preoccupation. Is it surprising that in an age of diet culture in extremis, we are more obsessed with food than ever?

I also propose we apply serious scrutiny to the healthy ideals to which we strive. The obsessive zeal with which so many track, quantify and regiment their food intake seems very far from healthy, in any true sense of the word. As someone whose bones will likely always bear the marks of anorexia, the irony of this strikes very close to home.

Diet culture is so mind-numbingly boring. That I am now awakened to this is one of the few good things to have come out of my illness. How much collective brain power, I wonder, is wasted counting calories? How much misspent anxiety and guilt is projected onto food, when eating is a basic need, as natural as breathing?

Although eating disorders are about much more than food and weight, they are chronic conditions, and I will probably always have to be careful. Given my history and genetic predisposition, I will never be able to trust myself to go on a diet. This, too, I consider a blessing. To have been thrown over the abyss means, I hope, that I will never again teeter on the edge. Anorexia has taken a great deal from me, but it has given me perspective.

So as we head into a new decade, and enter the season of fresh starts and rekindled gym memberships, my new year's resolutions this year are a little different. In 2020, I would like to fall in love with food again. I want to listen to my body, and to eat without fear, guilt or shame. This year, I don't want to count a single calorie, or track a single step. For me, these are big goals, but unlike my resolutions of previous years, if I achieve them, I think I just might be able to stick to them.

15 January 2020

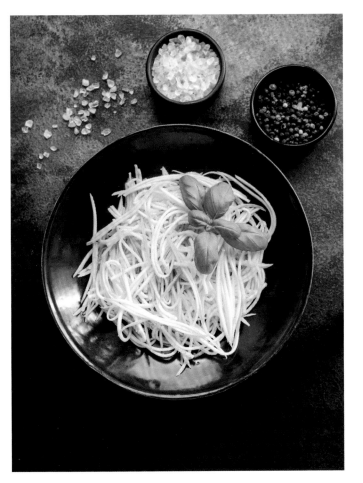

Anorexia is not what defines me; it is the way I fought to recover from the illness that does

Eating disorders are serious mental illnesses that involve disordered eating behaviour. This might mean limiting the amount of food eaten, eating very large quantities of food at once, getting rid of food eaten through unhealthy means or a combination of these behaviours.

Eating disorders affect males and females of all ages, can cause serious harm and may be fatal – anorexia has the highest mortality rate of all mental illnesses. But even though they are serious illnesses, eating disorders are treatable

'M' is recovering from anorexia, a severe eating disorder that affects 1.6 million people in the UK and is one of the most challenging conditions to treat and recover from. She received treatment and support from our award-winning specialist eating disorder service Cotswold House, at the Warneford Hospital. This is her powerful story.

I am currently in my second year of university: something I would not have been able to say had I not started my recovery from anorexia.

My eating disorder began around September 2017, although it is difficult to pinpoint a time. I didn't recognise its onset, I didn't even have much knowledge or awareness of eating disorders, I didn't ever suspect it could happen to me.

All I knew was that I was very unhappy; I think that this manifested itself into my desire to control something in my life, to have a focus, and something that was mine. Although having a focus can be positive, my focus was not.

At the time, I had just started an art foundation course but was very unsure of what I really wanted to do having just finished my A Levels.

I believe this uncertainty in my life and the fear of having to make big decisions contributed to the beginning of the Anorexia. However, I think it was also a long time coming – I had felt very unhappy for a long time in school with a low sense of confidence and self-worth contributing to this.

In the September 2017, I had just left school and started a new art course, a new job, and my first (not very healthy) relationship. During this time, I felt inadequate and lonely which started my obsession to improve myself by means of – what I thought at the time was – eating extremely healthily and exercising more.

Initially it was eating all the typically healthy foods and exercising more often; this incrementally became eating less altogether and exercising whenever I could. My mum noticed it first and tried to communicate this to me, although I was truly in denial and didn't believe what she said. I was just trying to be healthy.

It became more and more obsessive, with more and more rules taking over my life. These rules stopped me from going out with my friends and family, from being able to think about anything other than food and exercise, and from being free to make flexible plans, among many other things.

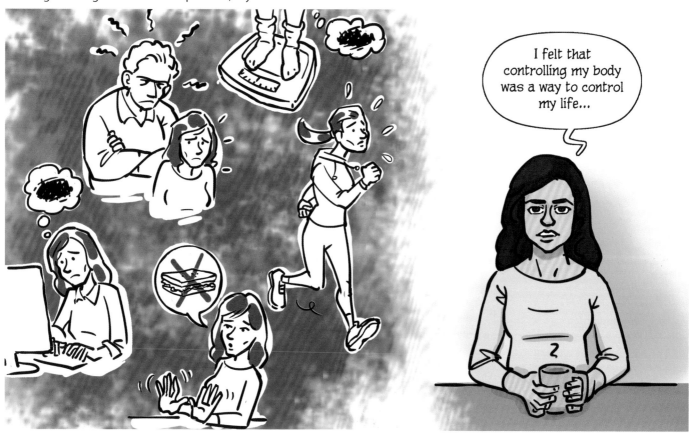

Bound by my rules

In May, I woke up one morning and felt overwhelmed with having to think so much about these rules controlling me. I couldn't contain it anymore and told my mum what was happening, even though I still didn't really understand it.

I went to the GPs that day and was told I needed to eat more and exercise less. Although this may be factually correct, this is not what someone with an eating disorder can do just by simply being told to. I did the reverse and throughout the year the behaviours became worse.

As a rule, I had to eat less and less every day and exercise more and more every day, even when I felt like I physically couldn't.

I could no longer laugh, or think creatively, or have the energy to talk. I was hurting my friends and my family, who pleaded with me to get better. People started to notice my appearance becoming worse, with some commenting on it, particularly my parents who were horrified by the way I was losing weight.

My mum and dad saw this happening and kept urging the GPs to help me access support – I owe so much to my parents for their unrelenting care. Eventually, around June, I was put in contact with a specialist eating disorder unit, where I was assessed and diagnosed with anorexia.

I was not at the stage, in terms of my weight, where admission to the inpatient unit was necessary. I was also told that the waiting list for receiving enhanced cognitive behaviour therapy (CBT-E) was over eight months, in which time I would have become even more ill.

Although I was given advice and resources to help change my behaviours, I refused to accept that I needed to, leading to a path of self-destruction. As my health was deteriorating to a dangerous level, I also felt a sense of achievement in being able to lose weight – a sign that I really needed help.

The eating disorder unit offered me a place on the inpatient ward which I said I would consider, although this would not have been a choice had I left it much longer. When I was at my worst my mum told me that if I did not eat, I would die, but I responded by saying that I would rather not eat.

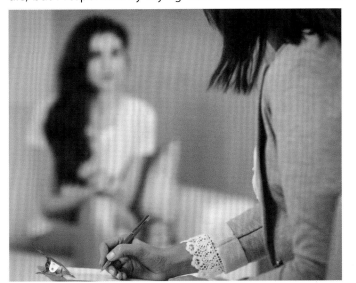

But this is what I am proud of – the work I put in to make these positive decisions every day.

Of course, this was not true, because this, in part, aided my decision to go into the inpatient eating disorder unit.

I went into the unit in August and was there until January 2018, where I was an inpatient until December and a day patient until January. It was the hardest process I have had to go through in my life, but also the most positively life changing one.

The people who cared for me there were some of the most amazing, motivational, and encouraging people I have ever met. I feel so grateful to the health care assistants, nurses, and doctors who looked after me every single day.

Whilst I was there, I received CBT-E once a week, which carried on until September 2018, just before I began university. The CBT-E I received was invaluable as I learnt so much, not only focusing on tackling the eating disorder but on recovering the important things in my life: my sense of self-worth, confidence, positive relationships, my interests and passions, and the balance between all of these things.

I slowly became physically healthier during my weight restoration journey and could start using my brain to do the CBT-E work and make sense of it all. It was a tough but crucial part of my recovery, and I feel so thankful for my therapist's support.

Starting university was scary – as it is for most people. I was doing well, but still mentally in the recovery process. Keeping consistency with what I ate and writing this down, alongside my thoughts and feelings, helped me so much to stay healthy and motivated to keep going.

It has not always been easy during university as routines sometimes change quickly and other people around me might eat erratically, as the typical university student does.

But keeping to my own routine and putting my needs first were very beneficial to me. I am now enjoying my second year of university, have made some amazing friends, am in the beginning of a positive relationship, and enjoy every moment with my family – all of which I could not achieve with Anorexia.

For me, recovery is a continuous journey where there are still times that are challenging and still, I must consciously strive to make the right decisions to continue onwards and upwards.

But this is what I am proud of – the work I put in to make these positive decisions every day.

I can now say that Anorexia is not what defines me; it is the way I have fought to recover from the illness, my connections to family and friends, and my choice to live by what truly makes me happy that defines me.

23 March 2020

Healthy eating is eating freely

Warning: I don't discuss specific behaviours or numbers in this article, but I do mention eating disorders and my own experience.

By Chloe

I'm going to eat 'healthier' and workout more. That's what I decided, over a year ago, with the sole motivation to gain some control during a stressful time in my life. Now, I'm in recovery from anorexia nervosa.

Subliminal messages encouraging weight loss, restrictive food habits, and excessive exercise allowed my disordered behaviours to be normalised as 'health-conscious' for a long time.

Given that recovery involves actively disobeying these messages by gaining weight, and that the survival response to malnourishment is to focus on nothing but food, it's no wonder I've developed a heightened awareness and hatred for diet talk. Whether it's relentless discussions of healthy eating at the dinner table, ads for weight-loss or 'guilt-free' products online, or a friend labelling entire food groups as good or bad – you've probably experienced diet culture.

Did you know that BMI, a common measure of health in medical settings, was invented by a mathematician and astronomer? In 1998 the USA, with no new scientific backing, moved the boundary for 'overweight' by two points. How reliable is this measurement, if it can be adjusted seemingly at random?

Did you know that your body has its own 'set point' and that this is a weight range to which it will return itself? Or that doctors in the USA have been known to be more reluctant in giving obese patients screening tests, and so these patients are 65% more likely to have a significant undiagnosed condition?

Neither did I. Until I had to recover from an eating disorder and undo years of fatphobic conditioning.

You've been told weight loss makes people happy. It doesn't. Companies, the celebrities they sponsor, and people profiting from that machine, will tell you whatever they need to, to make you pay up. But the truth? Trying to control our guilt by actively disobeying the nutritional needs of our bodies is as unhealthy as it gets.

During my disorder and subsequent weight loss, I was just following my rules. I was on my way to happiness, right? Well, as it turns out, wrong. My energy levels, bone density, organ functions, cognitive reasoning, ability to focus, think, laugh… they all took a hit.

This has led me to the conclusion that any diet - or 'lifestyle' as they're getting called now - is not going to let you lead

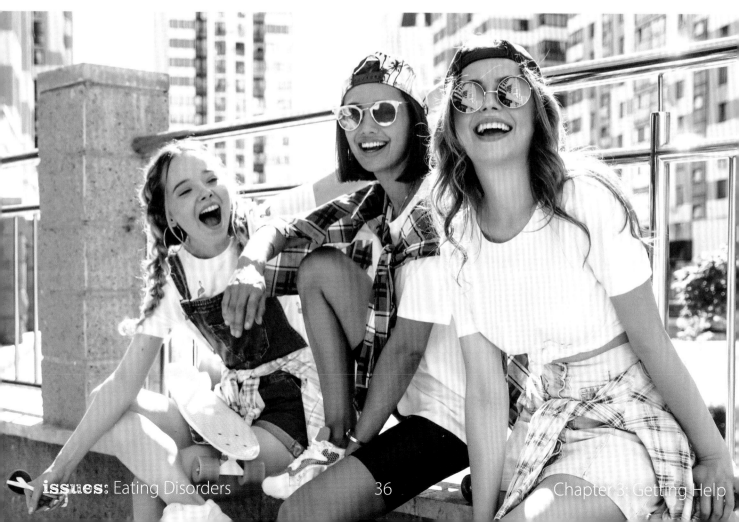

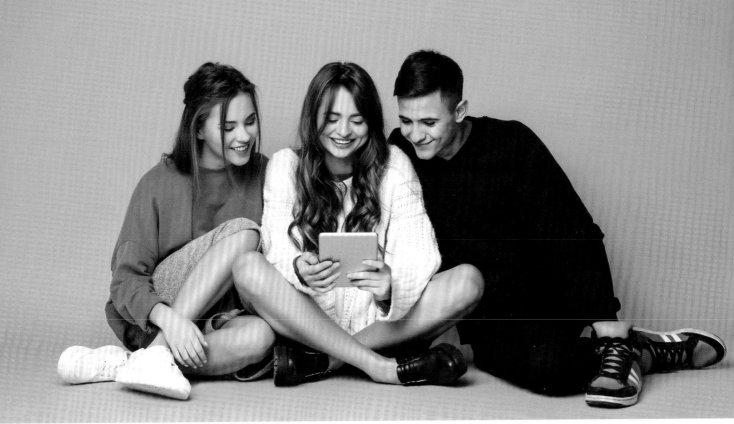

a happy, healthy life when it lets calories, gym time, or the number on the scale control you.

I would argue that the only way to achieve that freedom that we think comes from weight loss, is to disengage from the shame.

Here are some tips that I've found helpful for doing this:

- Don't comment on other people's food choices, and stand up for yourself if someone shames yours.

- Don't compliment weight loss, as this contributes to the idea that a bigger body is a problem to be solved. It could also be upsetting if the change has come from disordered habits, or lack of appetite due to any physical or mental illness.

- Don't engage in discussions about diets, workouts, or weight, and call others out on the damage they could be doing to others around them.

- Listen to all your cravings. You always have unconditional permission to eat what you truly enjoy, and by trusting and nourishing your body, you can put all your thoughts into things that really matter.

- Throw away the scales. Your relationship with gravity is unimportant.

- Unfollow any accounts focused on diet, fitness, or appearance, and shape your feed to be food and body-positive instead.

And above all, don't go on a damned diet in the new year! Health is freedom, and freedom is enjoying lunch with friends without worrying about the macros of your meal.

Please seek medical help if you think you could be suffering from disordered eating - you don't have to be a certain weight to be 'sick enough', nor do eating disorders have a specific 'look' in regards to size, race, gender, or age.

Thank you, Chloe for your thoughts on this important topic. As ever, we do encourage you to seek help if you think you might be suffering from any of the issues mentioned in this blog. We recommend you go to your local GP or visit Mind for further guidance and support.

16 January 2020

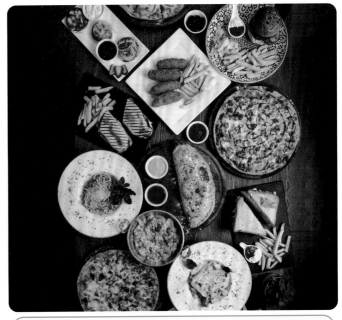

How can I stop an eating disorder relapse?

Dipping back into old, problematic behaviours can suck when you're in recovery for an eating disorder but relapses are common and are nothing to be ashamed of.

What is a relapse?

A relapse is when a person in recovery declines after a period of improvement. With an eating disorder this can mean that disordered thoughts and behaviours start to return.

What are the warning signs?

The warning signs of a relapse include:

- **Dishonesty:** If you're starting to bargain with yourself when it comes to eating patterns or you're beginning to twist the truth to those around you then you may be trying to rationalise disordered thoughts.

- **Feeling guilty:** Eating disorders can often stem from negative feelings towards yourself, your situation and what you're eating. A big part of recovery is learning how to deal with these negative thought patterns. If you are struggling, speak to your GP, therapist or whoever is supporting your recovery.

- **Isolation:** Starting to feel depressed or withdrawn from those around you is a sign that you may need extra help.

- **Changing eating habits:** Eating habits are a big part of eating disorders and recovery. If you're dipping back into old routines then there may be a problem. If you're supporting a loved one through recovery then this is something more obvious to look out for.

Why does it happen?

Relapses are a normal and expected part of recovery so don't feel ashamed if you experience them. Being in recovery for an eating disorder is tough work. It's unlikely that you'll be able to stay on one straight path as there are always ups and downs.

Circumstances in your life can change or you may experience unavoidable triggers. There are many reasons why someone may begin to dip again into patterns of an eating disorder.

Can you prevent a relapse?

Although it can be hard to predict if and when you may relapse there are a few steps you can take alongside any professional treatment you're receiving:

Set ACHIEVABLE goals: If we could put 'ACHIEVABLE' in shiny, glittering lights then we would. It's super important to have goals in recovery. Dreaming big is wonderful but sometimes having goals that are too big will only put pressure on you and make it harder for you in the long run. Setting achievable goals, even something as simple as making sure to eat breakfast every day, ensures you can succeed more often.

Write down your possible triggers: Noting down triggers can make you feel more in control and prepared for any future confrontation with them. Your triggers may feel overwhelming but it is important to be aware of them so you can seek help, from your doctor or therapist, to overcome them.

Have a plan in place with family and friends: If you prepare for a relapse with family and friends in advance it will make sure they know what to do if it happens and will know how to spot the warning signs. They could prepare how they'll speak to you about it, have some distraction ideas ready or make a list of contact numbers and websites for support.

Remind yourself of your progress: Self care is important no matter who you are or what you're going through, but if you are experiencing an eating disorder relapse it is an essential part of your recovery. Remind yourself of your progress by talking about it with someone close to you, make a happy box full of comforting memories or simply reflect on one good thing every day. This will keep you positive and motivated.

Stay positive on bad days: Looking after yourself is even more important on those bad days you will inevitably have. Take a chill day, spend time with good friends and treat yourself especially well. Don't let your negative thoughts spiral.

Remember that relapsing is nothing to be ashamed of and it can be a normal part of the recovery process. By being aware and prepared for the possibility of a relapse you'll make it easier to get back on track. If you need any more information visit Beat's website.

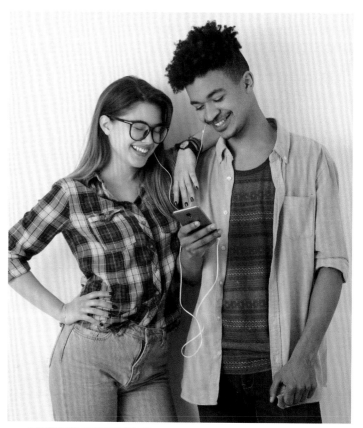

Where can I find help?

Below are some telephone numbers, email addresses and websites of agencies or charities that can offer support or advice if you, or someone you know, needs it.

Your GP or local NHS eating disorder team can provide help and support.

Childline
0800 1111
childline.org.uk

Young Minds
85258 (Crisis Messenger for young people – text the letters YM)
youngminds.org.uk

The Mix
themix.org.uk

Samaritans
116 123 (freephone)
jo@samaritans.org

Anorexia and Bulimia Care (ABC)
03000 11 12 13
anorexiabulimiacare.org.uk

Beat
0808 801 0677 (adult helpline)
0808 801 0711 (youthline)
0808 801 0811 (studentline)
beateatingdisorders.org.uk

National Centre for Eating Disorders
0845 838 2040
www.eating-disorders.org.uk

Overeaters Anonymous Great Britain
oagb.org.uk

SEED
01482 718130
www.seedeatingdisorders.org.uk

Weight Concern
www.weightconcern.org.uk

Weight Wise
www.bdaweightwise.com

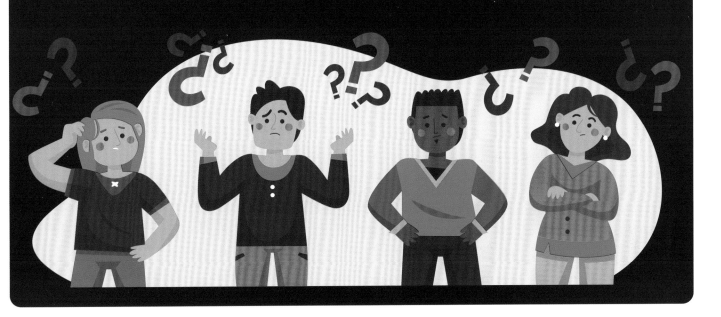

Key Facts

- Approximately 1.25 million people in the UK have an eating disorder. (Page 3)

- OSFED (other specified feeding or eating disorder) is the most common disorder, followed by binge eating disorder and then bulimia. Anorexia is the least common. (Page 3)

- Up to 6.4% of the population showing signs of developing an eating disorder. (Page 4)

- More than one in four young women have a potential eating disorder (Page 8)

- Four per cent said anxieties about food impinged their ability to work, carry out personal responsibilities or have a social life. (Page 8)

- Research found 27 per cent of men and 29 per cent of women were obese in 2019 — far higher than the 14 per cent of men and 17 per cent of women in 1994. (Page 8)

- The amount of adults with diabetes has trebled in the last 25 years - rising from three per cent of men and two per cent of women in 1994 to nine per cent and six per cent respectively in 2019. (Page 8)

- It is estimated that between 10% and 25% of those with an eating disorder are men. (Page 9)

- Women were more likely than men to screen positive for a possible eating disorder (19% and 13%, respectively). (Page 9)

- Among women, prevalence was highest in those aged under 35 (28% of those aged 16 to 24, 27% aged 25 to 34). (Page 9)

- Women were more likely than men to report that their feelings about food had a significant negative impact on their lives. (Page 10)

- Adults who screened positive for a possible eating disorder were more likely to have seen a GP in the last 12 months than adults who did not screen positive. (Page 10)

- One in five women in England may have an eating disorder. (Page 12)

- The number of urgent referrals for children and young people starting treatment in the community has reached an all-time high. (Page 12)

- Studies suggest that risk of mortality for males with eating disorders is higher than it is for females. (Page 15)

- 90% of teenage boys exercise with the purpose of bulking up. (Page 15)

- 15,558 people in Wales were diagnosed as having eating disorders between 1990 and 2017. (Page 16)

- One community support group, Talking Eating Disorders Liverpool (TEDS), says it has seen around a 50% increase in the number of adults and children seeking help. (Page 26)

- Beat, a national charity for people with eating disorders, has seen an 81 per cent increase in contact across all Helpline channels. This includes a 125 per cent rise in social media contact and a 115 per cent surge in online group attendance. (Page 31)

- Anorexia, a severe eating disorder, affects 1.6 million people in the UK. (Page 34)

Anorexia athletica

An eating disorder and mental health condition that involves excessively exercising in order to lose weight.

Anorexia nervosa

An eating disorder and mental health condition that involves an immoderate restriction on food intake.

Binge eating disorder

An eating disorder where a person feels compelled to consume large quantities of food in a short period of time, often when they are not hungry.

BMI (body mass index)

An abbreviation which stands for 'body mass index' and is used to determine whether an individual's weight is in proportion to their height. If a person's BMI is below 18.5 they are usually seen as being underweight. If a person has a BMI greater than or equal to 25, they are classed as overweight and a BMI of 30 and over is obese. As BMI is the same for both sexes and adults of all ages, it provides the most useful population-level measure of overweight and obesity. However, it should be considered a rough guide because it may not correspond to the same degree of 'fatness' in different individuals (e.g. a body builder could have a BMI of 30 but would not be obese because their weight would be primarily muscle rather than fat).

Body dysmorphic disorder (BDD)

A mental health condition where a person is preoccupied with their appearance which they believe has many flaws. These perceived flaws are often unnoticeable to others.

Body image

Body image is the subjective sense we have of our appearance and the experience of our physical embodiment. It is an individual's perception of what they look like or how they should look. It can be influenced by personal memory along with external sources such as the media and comments made by other people.

Bulimia nervosa

An eating disorder and mental health condition that involves excessive food consumption followed by actions such as vomiting or the use of laxatives to compensate for their food intake.

Diabulimia

An eating disorder in which people with Type 1 diabetes deliberately give themselves less insulin than they need in order to lose weight.

Diet

The variety of food and drink that someone eats on a regular basis. The phrase `on a diet` is also often used to refer to a period of controlling what one eats while trying to lose weight.

Disordered eating

A term used to describe eating habits that can be considered `irregular' but do not warrant diagnosis as anorexia or bulimia nervosa.

Eating disorder

A term used to describe a range of psychological disorders that involve disturbed eating habits such as anorexia or bulimia nervosa.

Faddy eating

Similar to fussy eating; often involves the exclusion or avoidance of certain foods for no discernible reason.

Malnutrition

Malnutrition essentially means 'poor nutrition'. There are two types of malnutrition: undernutrition (when a person's diet is lacking in nutrients and sustenance they need) and overnutrition (when a person's diet is getting far too many nutrients for the body to cope with). Malnutrition can affect anybody, although it tends to be more common in developing countries where there are shortages of food.

Orthorexia nervosa

An eating disorder and mental health condition characterised by an extreme avoidance of food that the sufferer considers to be unhealthy.

Pica

A disorder that involves the consumption of non-nutritive substances such as dirt, hair or sand.

Size-zero

A term referring to U.S. clothing, size-zero is equivalent to a UK size-four. In order to fit into size-zero clothing an individual must have the waist measurement of 23 inches which is the average waist size of an eight-year-old.

Activities

Brainstorm

- Brainstorm what you know about eating disorders:

  - What are some of the different types of eating disorder?

  - Who is at risk of suffering from an eating disorder?

  - Why might someone develop an eating disorder?

  - What is the difference between an eating disorder and disordered eating?

  - What do you think may be common misperceptions of a person who has an eating disorder?

- Make a mind map on your relationship with food. Include the things that you enjoy or dislike about food and eating.

Design

- Choose an article from this topic and create an illustration to highlight its key themes.

- Create a leaflet explaining the signs and symptoms of eating disorders.

- Design a leaflet for young people to seek support if they have a friend who they think might be suffering from an eating disorder.

- Choose an article from this book and design a poster to show the key points from the article.

- Using the 'Where can I find help?' page in this book, design a poster for one of the organisations and include their contact details.

Oral

- Eating disorders are made worse by celebrities and social media. Debate this statement as a class, with half arguing in favour and half arguing against.

- Choose an illustration from this topic and, in pairs, discuss what the artist was trying to show with their cartoon.

- In pairs, discuss the following questions: What is disordered eating? How does it relate to eating disorders?

Reading/Writing

- Write an open letter to high-street clothes shops, imploring them to stop using ultra-thin mannequins in their shop windows. Make sure to include persuasive language.

- Read the article 'I'm recovering from an eating disorder' and write a letter or email to a celebrity that promotes diet products or alters their images and explain why you think that is damaging to their fans.

- Imagine that you are an Agony Aunt/Uncle who has received a letter from friend of someone who they think has an eating disorder. What advice would you give to them?

- Choose one of the articles in this book and write a short summary of the article and three key facts.

- Using the articles from Chapter 3: Getting Help, write a list of tips for someone who may be experiencing disordered eating to help them recover and develop a healthy relationship with food.

Index

Acknowledgements

The publisher is grateful for permission to reproduce the material in this book. While every care has been taken to trace and acknowledge copyright, the publisher tenders its apology for any accidental infringement or where copyright has proved untraceable. The publisher would be pleased to come to a suitable arrangement in any such case with the rightful owner.

The material reproduced in ISSUES books is provided as an educational resource only. The views, opinions and information contained within reprinted material in ISSUES books do not necessarily represent those of Independence Educational Publishers and its employees.

Images

Cover image courtesy of iStock. All other images courtesy of Freepik Pixabay and Unsplash.

Illustrations

Simon Kneebone: pages 4, 15 & 29. Angelo Madrid: pages 6, 17 & 34.

Additional acknowledgements

With thanks to the Independence team: Shelley Baldry, Danielle Lobban, Jackie Staines and Jan Sunderland.

Tracy Biram

Cambridge, May 2021